Let's Communicate, Breaking the Cycle of Non-communication

by

Dee Frances

DDDD Publications
9715 Foster Ste A
St. Louis Mo 63114

Printed in the U.S.A.

INTRODUCTION

THIS BOOK IS WRITTEN IN THE FIRST PERSON AND CONTAINS PERSONAL EXPERIENCES OF IT'S AUTHOR, DEE FRANCES. Dee has endeavored to keep illustrations to the types of things which probably go on in most families. The essence of this text is to help people see that the so called small things, are a vast part of the

nonsensical - non - system of things that when understood are a system of illogical, logic which has recently been labeled as dysfunction. To Survive this system without being insane our thinking pattern adapted to and around the system of non- communication to believe we are communicating.

Breaking the cycle of Non- communication is the strength to say:

"I'm not embarrassed to talk to others about my feelings or my problems. I know that the better the family the freer they are to ask the opinions of others, knowing that we can use part or all, or none of that information, our choice, as we feel it will work in our lives."

Breaking the cycle of non- communication means:

"I fully accept, "no man is an island," or woman either. Sharing with others builds love and trust in the world around us.

HOW TO USE THIS BOOK

You are certainly free to skip any section that you feel, you don't need, however I recommend reading from cover to cover, to gain better understanding of the world around you. We certainly hope that you are one of those fortunate persons, who has never been abused, but which ever the case your heart and love for mankind will grow by staying with all the material.

HOWEVER

If you are extremely busy, I suggest the following chapters be read first, then work on using this skills to see the quality of your life and your family's lives vastly improve. Than come back to the rest of this book for further insights.

Now for the chapters: Accurate Communication, Boundaries, Verbal Leverage, Fighting with Dignity, and True Autonomy.

Please send your comments to:DDDD Publications 9715 Foster Ste. A St. Louis Mo 63114 or see our web site @ www.a-rbooks.bigstep.com

Dee Frances

TABLE OF CONTENTS

CAN I HAVE THIS DANCE?

Can I have this dance? The dance of life awaits us. A functional life is like a beautiful waltz, hard work to learn, but lived with eloquence and dignity. When we see two people who waltz well the floor seems to clear in envy of their ability. Someone leads. Someone follows. Both an art to learn and carry out in a way that brings beauty to the dance as well as shows respect for ourself and our partner. Each part is as honorable as the other. Be it the lead for the male or the gracious art of skillfully following the lead while at the same time dancing our dance to show our individuality.

Dancing was always my way to release pent up feelings. Still today when I hurt, when I'm sick of it all, when I need a break, I dance. So to answer the question, can I have this dance? let's talk about breaking the cycle of dysfunction. The cycle that has kept us locked into a predictable and boring box step. A dysfunctional way of life that can be turned into a beautiful waltz is what we will be discussing throughout this book. Whenever you read the phrase, breaking the cycle of dysfunction, stop for just a moment and think about how those couples came to have the ability to dance their dance with skill and grace. We, too, can live our lives with the dignity of functionality.

I was dysfunctional. It is the delight of my life to be able to say with all certainty, "I am no longer dysfunctional." Yes, it is possible. This book is about how we got to be dysfunctional and better yet how do we break the cycle of dysfunction. How will we be able to say, "Can I have this dance?"

What is dysfunction? Codependency, a major outgrowth of dysfunction, it is known as a compulsive disorder. It could be defined as a compulsion to control in order to keep from being controlled.

First of all I'd like to address how we got to be dysfunctional. I came from generations of dysfunction, like the majority of us. Dysfunctional people produce dysfunctional children. When one or more people attempt to control a situation or another person's responses in any given situation the natural reaction of the person they are attempting to control is to resist that control. To resist control of our thoughts and feelings is a natural reaction to their attempt to control those same thoughts and feelings. Result: more dysfunction. Our dysfunction has become a natural way to protect ourselves from their dysfunction.

Other compulsive disorders like alcoholism, workaholism, foodaholism, perfectionism, rageaholism are all outgrowths of dysfunction. Each compulsive disorder that enters the picture on either parties end will complicate and make our dysfunction harder from which to break free.

Family situations that count on a child or the children to carry the responsibilities of the adults have the effect on the child's feeling that he or she is responsible for the actions of the adults. When a parent comes to rely on a child to be their problem solver or take on the role that a neglectful or absentee spouse is not filling the child is thus being used by the parent to fill the emotional needs of the parent. The child can never fill the needs that adults count on other adults to fill because they lack the life experience and knowledge of how things work in relationships. The entire system has set the child up for constant frustration. Despise all his or her hard work they will never be able to make mom or dad happy. They will never be able to clean like mom, or cook like mom, or work like dad. The child now emotionally freezes at their current age level. They cannot progress on with life. Their life is now caught up in surviving a system which has overburdened and destroyed their one most precious possession, their childhood. It is gone. In healing from dysfunction we will learn how to reclaim pieces of our childhood, draw them to our hearts, cherish the things from our inner true self that we held on to, the things that our child found so dear that today they are still within us speaking out to be heard. This book is about learning how to listen to your inner child. The child that you were. How to validate your child until she/he feels warm and secure. I believe the following poem describes the blessings we find when we are able to take care of our innermost needs.

MY BLESSING

My child inside is happy now,
she speaks for all to hear.

My child inside is happy now,
she whispers in my ear.

She snuggles down with warm delight,
nurtured and fulfilled.
blessed and forgiven,
she'll speak to me still.

From Poems and Growth from me to me by Dee Frances

BAGGAGE

I believe that the proper separation of baggage is the key ingredient in healing from dysfunction. As I considered reading materials what I kept seeing no matter what aspect of dysfunction or healing the author spoke of was, do not take the responsibility for the thoughts, feelings, actions, and reactions of others. I believe what they do they do. What I do I do. Do not be embarrassed for others. I will be embarrassed if my actions were inappropriate to the situation. I can be embarrassed long enough to learn to look for more appropriate ways to act under similar situations. But I will not be embarrassed over what others do. I will not lie for them because of my embarrassment. I need not take on any of the responsibility for their actions nor will I take on embarrassment about what I think others must think of me now because I am, their sister, their wife, or their mother, or whatever the relationship happens to be.

The best definition I can give of baggage is; each of us has choices. The things that happen as a result of their choices are their baggage. The things that happen as a result of my choices are my baggage.

As a child I did not realize there were sometimes more choices available to me than I was aware. Dysfunctional adults, those that are struck at a child's level are still unaware of many of life's choices. Thus comes the most dysfunctional phrase I know. "They left me no choice." The word, "they," indicating the dysfunctional person does not accept the responsibility for their own choice and "left me no choice,' stemming from the fact that dysfunctional persons think in all or nothing terms. It is this or that. Black or white. That are no shades of gray. There is nothing between this and that. There is only this or that.

Separation of baggage is difficult to learn even for adults. As children with no guidance from those who knew how to separate baggage we failed to learn this skill properly. We have all heard of Robert Fulcrum's book Everything I Needed to Know I Learned in Kindergarten, but I believe that for those of us who came from the roots of dysfunction it would be more accurate to say, Everything I Needed to Know, I Had to Figure Out.

With the above in mind I would like to list some to the things I figured out in regards to the subject of baggage. This list is included in my book 1475 Conclusions of a Healing Codependent.

When I start to separate baggage I start the healing process.

Separating baggage allows me to be grieve my losses.

Separating baggage allows me to be realistic about my losses.

When I properly separate baggage I have less loses then when I am taking the blame for others, carrying their baggage as well as mine. Even though sometimes it feels like my losses are more.

When we start to separate baggage we will be angry. Angry that they put their guilts on us. Angry we let them.

Others will change only when they want, if they don't it is their baggage.

Just because someone perceives me a certain way does not mean that is what I am. I need not take the responsibility, baggage, for their thoughts or actions.

I cannot and will not deal with your feelings.

I will take responsibility for my own thoughts, feelings, actions, and reactions.

When I separate baggage I will not let others put their guilts on me.

As we separate baggage we will become more and more secure.

When we Properly separate baggage we can establish a start to good communication. I can now say, "When you did...... I felt,......." instead of "Do you know what you did to me?" We are now able to know which part was them and which part is us.

If I deny my right to my thoughts, feelings, needs, and desires that is my fault, my baggage.

If I feel miserable when others criticize me, I have taken the blame for their perceptions and my weak points.

I have come to understand that many of my perceptions were correct. I failed myself when I turned those negative things on myself. I faulted myself because of the actions of others. I did not know how to separate baggage.

I am responsible only for making myself happy. I can role model to others a healthy relationship with myself. If they are interested in being truly happy from within and not being dependent on others for their happiness I can help by saying, "This worked for me....." they can copy my example if and when they choose.

Not everyone cares about the other person's feelings, it is my baggage to protect myself from their lack of caring.

I can care about your feelings without taking responsibility for them.

These are but a few of the conclusions I was able to draw that enabled myself to have the power I needed to work my way through recovery.

STARTING THE ROAD OF RECOVERY

I believe I started down the road of recovery when I was thirteen years old. This road was opened up to me by the one that was protecting me. One traumatic night I laid in bed weeping from my heart. How could I take it? There's no way out? I prayed for His protection, His guidance. But only after I earnestly begged to die. I could not see how I could maintain my sanity. What came over me at that time was a feeling that I would come to know several more times in my life. I would be struck with not a new thought but a new thought process. It was not really me guiding this thing. I came to know that night that I would survive. I would survive in charge of my soul. They could only crush it if I let them. It's my soul. I will survive in charge of my soul. And I did.

Since that time I have learned that this was the heart of dysfunction. My controlling child had completely taken over to protect my hurting self so that I could survive until the day that my God would again lead me. This time in the search to find the soul that had not been crushed. It had only been buried. I had become codependent. I had not become dead. I can heal from codependency. I cannot heal from dead. Again my God has not let me down.

From this time on I began, at least some of the time, to be able to separate some things into this was me and this is you. Although I worked hard to make things right in the home, I wanted very much to protect my mother and my sisters, but I knew that some of the things they did were them. I tried to fix in my efforts to help them so they could see how useless these types of actions were and are. These were my efforts to control.

I started the road of recovery in the sense that I knew that I had to take care of myself. I started my road of recovery because I was able in some cases to distinguish what they did from what I did. That I was not responsible for....... I started my road of recovery because I was able to determine in my own mind what I wanted to copy and what I knew that I would do different with my life.

All of these things are essential ingredients in breaking the cycle of dysfunction. How it also contributed to my dysfunction I connected with what Timmen Cermak describes in his book A Time to Heal. I had begun to identify what I was by what I was not. If they were out of control, I could be in control. If they were angry. I was nice. If they drink, I don't. If they...... I don't. Whatever they were, I was not. We are still being controlled by what they are or were. We are being controlled in our efforts to control. I can show them that I'm not a..... I'm not like that. I can rise above this...... Truth being we cannot rise above this. We take it with us wherever we go until the day that we begin to separate baggage. Learning enough about how to go about it that we will be able not to improve on separating baggage but we will learn the joy of baggage separation. We will come to do it so well, without thought, that no one can ever guilt trip us again. (This comes with time and practice.)

Starting down the road of recovery means we accept that we as a person deserve to be validated. Some of this validation comes about by knowing others who have lived through the same type of circumstances have the same types of feelings and/or reactions we have had. The differences in us and them may be that another person has acted on things that on which we have chosen not to act. An example of this would be in the case of wanting vengeance on another. Some choose to act in a vengeful way. I choose not to...... In my days of dysfunction I chose not to, "return evil for evil," today I choose not to, "return evil for evil," however, at this point in time, I know that I can protect myself from abuse and other peoples dysfunction without vengeance. I think the greatest thing I have learned is that I can take care of me without hurting you.

The feelings we have experienced were a normal response to abnormal behaviors. When we come to understand we fall within the range of normal human feelings we are starting our road to recovery. Even in the case of our own wrongdoings we can learn the art of self acceptance by knowing and applying this motto to our lives; "what I did may not be right but I now know it was a normal reaction to the circumstances I had to live with at that time."

This is what is involved in the fine art of learning how to let go. Learning how to forgive ourselves. I know where I was wrong. I regret my wrongs. I sincerely want to work on me. Working on me means I must learn how to separate baggage appropriately. I will not accept the shame and guilt associated with your actions. I will accept total responsibility for my actions and reactions. I am learning to release my fear of making mistakes.

Dysfunction requires that we do not make mistakes. In our dysfunctional families we learned it was dangerous to make mistakes. At the very least, we learned we would be humiliated and degraded for the smallest of errors. In the process of breaking the cycle of dysfunction we are learning there are others who do accept us as a good and decent person even when we make mistakes. When we accept there are accepting loving people in this world, people who are not afraid to reach out to another heart, we also begin to accept we are loved by them. This may be strange and frightening at the time as we are not accustomed to acceptance.

This leads me to the point in time where I again am aware of another step taken down the road of recovery. My husband and I had been married a few months. I had gotten a bargain on a large three pound jar of jelly. I reached for it with one hand. Of course, I dropped it. It went all through the breakfast and down the front of the stove. I gasped. I shook. I shook some more. My bewildered husband kept asking, "what's wrong?" I not being able to reply stood there and shook. He approached saying, "It's only jelly. Don't worry about it." He held me until I calmed down. As I wept on his shoulder my inner self was screaming with delight, "This is it! This is it! This is what I have been looking for!" For the next couple of weeks I think I must have asked at least daily, "how come you didn't scream at me when I dropped the jelly?" His reply always was, "Nobody screams at people for dropping the jelly. You just don't do that." But although I did not tell him so, I knew that people do scream at you, hit you, belittle and abuse over dropped jars of jelly. It was at this time that I began to get angry. Angry at my family of origin. I knew my husband loved me. I felt it. My anger at my family arose from this question, "This is how people are supposed to treat other people. My husband says people don't scream over a broken jar of jelly because you love me. This is love. Why? Why couldn't the other people in my life that claimed love for me do this? Did they love me? It didn't feel like love? Was it?"

HOW DO WE KNOW IF WE ARE DYSFUNCTIONAL?

Can we say no? Can we say No without guilt? Are the things that go wrong others people's fault? Do we feel guilty for being angry? Do we only feel safe when we are angry? Can we talk to others about our feelings? Do we think we know what others think about us? Do we worry about what others think when we mess up? Do we worry about what others think of us when our loved ones mess up? Do we need to keep our distance in a relationship to keep from being hurt? Do we allow ourselves to be in a relationship? Does each relationship hurt more than the last relationship? Do we tolerate an abusive relationship just so we won't be alone? Do we think they (the opposite sex) are all like that, I might as well stay? Do we eat to feel better? Do we drink to feel better? Do we think our way through our problems rather than feel what we need to feel? Do we dump our problems on others to handle? Do we expect ourselves to fail? Do we not finish projects rather than admit that we fear we cannot do them? Do we get sick when we are angry? Do needy people need us? Do we constantly over work or over commit? Do we let others pressure us into things we do not want to do? Are we afraid of not be wanted? Do I believe tears are weakness? Do I believe that I must always put others before myself? Must I be tough? Do I believe to be sad is weakness? Do I feel guilty if my thoughts and feelings are different than the thoughts and feelings of those I care about? Do we go to doctors who tell us we are fine then we go to another doctor because the first was incompetent? Are we involved with the need for tranquilizers? Do we have to tell ourselves things will be better tomorrow to get through today on a regular bases? Are we happy only when things are going well? Do we have to please others to be happy only to find out we are not happy? Do we believe others will not be there for us? When unpleasant things happen do we say or think, 'it's been that way all my life why should it change now?' Do we equate love with pain and unhappiness? Do we check on others? Do we use up all our energy to help others only to find we receive no help? Could we tell hair raising tales? Do we carry great disappointment? Do we fear what will happen to us if we are not in charge, control? Can we relax and just let things happen? Do we fear letting things happen without our hand in the matter?

Have we come to know how things should be? Are we advice givers? Do we dominate? Do we manipulate? Do we carefully pick our words to get the response for which we hope? Do we get upset when our advice is not taken? Do we feel we are not taken seriously? Is it difficult to get to the point in our conversations? Do we repeat ourselves because we are never sure we are understood? Do we say differently than we mean? (saying yes when we want to say no.) Do we lie to cover our actions or the actions of others? Do we feel we have the right to say, no? Do we tell people what we will not stand for only to find they do it anyway, then we tell them again, but the cycle keeps going? Do we complain about how others treat us but don't know how to change it? Are we frequently disappointed because we find we trusted an untrustable person? Are we afraid of anger? Are we ashamed of our background? Do we feel pity for our parents? Do we use our anger to punish those who hurt us? Do we wish our sex partner would fade away or die? Do we make excuses not to have sex? Do we not understand why we don't enjoy sex? Do we use sex as our way to feel good? Do we have to force ourselves to have sex when we really don't want sex? Is sex routine? Are we overly responsible? Do we put our responsibilities on others? Are we other peoples' victim? Are we manipulated by other peoples tears? Do we manipulate by use of tears? Do we continually sacrifice our happiness for others? Do we use violence to control others? Have we reached the point that nothing is worth the effort needed to carry it out? Do we feel suicidal?

If we have answered yes to any of these questions we are to some degree dysfunctional. Dysfunction like anything else in life comes in varying stages. The more questions we answered yes to the more severe the dysfunction. At one time I would have answered yes to almost all or the above, however, today I would answer NO to all of the above. What is it that will make the difference between the functional and the dysfunctional? Several main ingredients are;

1. I have no fear of any of my feelings. I know I have learned to act appropriately with each type of feeling I have.

2. I have no shame over my background. I know that the things that happened to me

were events. They are not me. I know my feelings are not my personality. Every personality has anger, sadness, happiness, guilt, and excitement. I believe my personality is what I have chosen to do about my feelings. I can hang onto them. I can choose to change them. I can let go of the things that hurt me. I can talk about them. The choices are mine.

3. I do not get embarrassed over the actions of others.

4. I am comfortable talking about my feelings in appropriate places and with trustable people. I do not expect everyone to be there for me. I do not expect no one to be there for me.

5. I do not have to be in charge to protect myself from the things that might happen. I can relax and let things happen. I do not have to make them happen a certain way to know that I am safe.

6. I can say no without guilt.

7. I can make a change in plans without feeling I must explain to others why?

8. I have learned how to listen, not just talk.

9. I laugh not to cover my sadness but because I have true joy of heart.

10. I do not eat to feel good.

11. I need not laugh to cover my embarrassment. I laugh if and when I want to laugh.

12. I have learned, I can care about others and take care of myself at the same time.

13. I do not have to get everything right. I have learned, I can't do everything right. I

don't do everything wrong. I can relax and enjoy the beauty of my averageness.

14. I have seen and felt the joy of seeing my family join with me in recovery. Just today my three year old grandson went with us to a religious meeting. We promised him if he was very quiet he could have the second half of a candy bar he had purchased with his own money. When we returned home my seventeen year old son had eaten it. My son-in-law stopped by to give the boy a hug good night. He was told that Matt had eaten Lucas's candy. Dad said, "Did you tell him how you feel about that?" Lucas went into the room where my son was watching T.V. and said, "Uncle Matt I have to tell you how I feel. You ate my candy bar." ----- "I did."------- "Well, you knew it wasn't yours. You knew it was mine." ------ "Well, I did not know it was yours, Lucas." ------- "You knew it was not yours. I don't like this thing you did." Matt's reply, "I'm sorry Lucas. I will buy you some candy when I get my check." Lucas then replied, "Okay, this time. I don't like this thing you did."

I have included this small, but important example because this is functional at it's best. This is a three year old who was allowed by his father and all other adults in the family to talk about why he was angry. Just as important the seventeen year old listened, apologized, and offered what he could to make amends.

Because he is allowed to express his feelings Lucas at the tender age of three also knows there is a right way and a wrong way to express his needs. He did not scream, throw things, or call names. He simply said he did not like the thing his uncle Matt did.

The biggest part of being functional is having the ability to address the thing that was done. We do not degrade the quality of the person because a bad decision was made. We can take joy into our hearts knowing that if a healthy three year old child possesses these skills then we too can acquire these same abilities as we learn to break our cycle of dysfunction.

We become capable of breaking the cycle of dysfunction as we become less and less shame based. We become less and less shame based as we break the cycle of dysfunction. Recovery is a paradox. Recovery is full of paradoxes. I believe we start recovery by acting functional whether or not we feel functional. We learn not to control even though we feel like controlling. We learn not to check on someone even though we feel like checking on them. We learn to say, "When you walk out of the room when I'm talking I get nervous. I feel you must not care about what I'm saying." We do this even though we feel like saying, "You make me nuts. You walk out of the room. You are inconsiderate. Stop it!"

The above illustrates that to break the cycle of dysfunction we first must act functionally. We must prime the pump. We learn to say, "I'm angry because....." as we get more and more accustomed to phrasing our statements of conversation in an appropriate way we also learn we can express even feelings of anger without a battle. We then become less afraid of confrontation. The less we fear confrontation the more we will be able to say no when someone asks us to do something for which we do not have the time or would prefer not to do for any reason, maybe this thing crosses one of my boundaries. Each of these steps enables or empowers us to grow. Each of these steps empowers us to empower ourselves. We do so by finding the delight and strength of person that comes our way by putting each of these small steps into practice. In a later chapter we will discuss in more detail examples of functional verses dysfunctional conversations.

Codependency is the major outgrowth of dysfunction. Codependency can best be defined as a state of being wherein the person does not feel free to express their wants or needs. As a codependent I felt guilty if my thoughts and feelings were different than those of the people that I cared about. This I see as a direct result of statements that our subconscious recorded, as if a tape recorder, many years ago in our childhoods. Children learn to feel ashamed of their ideas when they eagerly share an idea with an adult only to be told, "Where did you ever get an idea like that?" or, "Your head must be on loose." Other popular phrases would be, "What an idiot." "Your so stupid," "That's the stupidest thing I ever heard." "Don't even bother me." All these are an attempt to belittle and control the child so the parents will always have the upper hand, control.

Each family member has now become ashamed of their family unit. Even when children have not witnessed a more civil standard of conduct between people something inside their heart tells them that their family is different. Their family business must remain silent in order for each family member not to be shamed in public. Each family member without talking to other family members now takes whatever steps their personality deems necessary to protect the family from disclosure. Or the opposite may be true. One or sometimes more family members may react as a rebel. They have become the family scapegoat. Everything that goes wrong is blamed on this person and it seems to be so as each of their rebellious actions brings more shame on this family. Other family members must now work harder to cover family and personal shame. The rebel in turn must act out more so in order to try to bring attention to the realities of dysfunction and/or abuse. The cycle of dysfunction and it's consequences stage has been set. The players have been assigned their perspective roles. Each person locks into a specific role to be carried out for the rest of their lives, unless somewhere in the process they find their road of recovery. When they do they will be met with opposition, anger, and manipulations. Other family members will enact the phrase, "No family member is allowed to be healthier than the sickest family member." To do otherwise is, as the family sees it, the ultimate betrayal of parents and family.

Like it or not each family member must now endeavor to be responsible for all other family members. Thus we learned how to control. It is easier for us to accept that we are responsible than to accept they are responsible. If we believe we are responsible there is hope of change. If we believe they are responsible and they do not change, we feel trapped, bound in a hopeless situation. If we believe that we are responsible for this or that then we have hope of changing the family picture. Maybe if I..... things will be better. If we believe that they are the one responsible we know we cannot change them thus we have no hope, no dreams of a brighter day. If I am responsible than I can...... and everything will be fine. The more we try to help the more we must help. If I do this they will need me. They will love me. I am loved. What human can be a happy well rounded person if we do not feel loved. Here note the key word is **feel.**

In the dysfunctional family chances are everyone loves everyone. No one is able to communicate their love to the others. No one knows how to listen in a way to validate the feelings of the others. Everyone in the family is trying to hold this family together. Everyone feels they are doing the largest share of the work. Everyone feels dumped on, and worse of all no one feels loved. Everyone is loved. Sad but true no one feels loved.

Because of the lack of communication and validation we feel shame over our feelings. If as a child I was angry and I express my anger only to be told, "You shouldn't feel that way. It's not nice," then I learn to feel shame when I have anger. I have learned anger is a natural and healthy response. Anger is our best protector. It enables us to say, "Stop, don't touch me." or "I need space so I can calm down. If I try to talk now I will end up saying something both of us will regret." Anger protects me from their verbal abuse. Anger expressed appropriately protects myself from verbally abusing others.

I have learned, God has anger. No, He is not an angry God. He is a Happy God. He is happy because He handles His anger appropriately. His anger is what is referred to as justifiable anger. Would you be angry if you could see all of the abuse and crime that is going on in the world. Yet His love for mankind is what motivates God to help even the abuser to sort and separate the things that have happened to them from what they are as a person. He will lead them down their path of recovery if only they reach for it.

When I learn any feeling I have has been felt by all people walking the earth or that have walked the earth I can relax. I need not feel shame if I am angry, sad, or happy. Yes, some of us have been shamed over laughing. Ridding ourselves or our personal shame throws away from us much of the misery we have carried. Let us illustrate how by explaining how shame turns into other negative feelings.

"Shame turns into rage. The rageaholic uses their rage to keep others at a distance. Others will not be able to get close enough to see their shame. This person feels safest when they demonstrate their anger.

Shame turns into indifference. We don't care. We are not shamed. Nothing matters anyway.

Shame turns into the need to control. If we can control we can prove to ourselves we are okay. See what I can do, with control comes power not shame.

Shame produces depression. Our shame is because we are not okay. How can we feel good about ourselves? We are not okay. We can't help but be depressed. Many dysfunctional people suffer chronic low grade depression, a constant sadness.

Shame produces confusion. We feel guilty. But my little inner voice said, "NO! NO! THAT'S NOT RIGHT! SOMETHING ISN'T RIGHT HERE! DO I REALLY BELIEVE THIS OR THAT? NO! THEY MUST THINK I'M STUPID!" Profile of Abuse by Dee Frances.

Shame basing also occurs when boundaries are violated. Boundaries will be discussed in great detail in a later chapter but for now let's define boundaries as an invisible fence. This is as far as I can let you go and still feel safe. I have the right and moral duty to myself not to let others cross my boundaries. At the same time I will not deliberately cross or step on your boundaries. If you begin to cross mine I will honor you by telling you, not abusing you. If I unknowingly step on your boundaries, please honor me by telling me how you feel. We can both then work toward respecting each others rights and feelings as a person different than ourselves.

When we deal directly with the issues which caused our shame we will then be releasing all the others affects shame has had upon us. We will deal with every feeling in a more appropriate way. We will now be able to work what is referred to as an honest recovery program. We are being honest about our abilities and our weakness. We will find the joy of being able to say with gladness of heart, "Good job. Job well done," to ourselves with no fear of guilt.

Removing Shame from our hearts removes the need for compulsive disorders. These include, alcoholism, drugs, compulsive overeating, compulsive under eating, gambling, sexaholism, thingaholism, workaholism, and shopaholism.

Shame and guilt are quite different. Learning from John Bradshaw's Bradshaw on: The Family the difference between guilt and shame I can now say , "Guilt always say's I've done something wrong." Shame felt; there is something wrong with me. f These words are from page two of his book. Upon reading this I was hooked. While Codependent No More started teaching me how to separate baggage, Bradshaw's book would teach me how my role in the family rooted me in the cycle of dysfunction. Better still his book showed me how I can use the things I used in dysfunction as part of my recovery. Yes, many of the skills I learned by being the family star would also be the skills I would use to my advantage in the course of recovery. In the course of recovery I would come to answer the most important questions of my life. Who am I? Did I know? How could I find out? You say codependency is a false self, what happened to the real me? I'm changing but I'm scared of the changes, what will be left when the controlling is gone? Will I like me? Will you like me? Is it going to be worth all this hard work?

WHO AM I?

The biggest error each dysfunctional person makes is that of ignoring our feelings for the sake of everyone else's feelings. When I do good to you, I am good! So I thought. The Karpman's drama triangle says we give until it hurts, then we persecute, then we become their victim. We have again and again rescued others from their consequences. By doing so we have enabled them to continue in whatever course they are pursuing. We fix their problem. They do not learn from their mistakes. They repeat. We repeat. The more we help them the more we resent them. The more we help others the less we know ourselves. We become so wrapped up in them and their problems we hardly stop to think about how we feel, what we need, or acknowledge that we have wants other than continually bailing the other person or persons out of trouble.

If we are living with an alcoholic or other compulsive person we watch over them and protect them from harms way. I would rescue out a sense of urgency to do something. Sometimes I rescued out of fear of what would happen if somebody did not do something. Other times we may rescue because we feel more capable of handling the situation than other parties involved.

All of the above adds up to carrying out the original role taken on in our original dysfunctional family. In order to break the cycle of dysfunction we need to learn how not to react to their actions. They act. We react. They react to our reaction. We react. They react. Someone, anyone in the process can stop the cycle of act, react, react some more. I can stop. Think. I can learn how not to react to their actions or reactions. When I learn how not to react to whatever is going on with them I am giving up being controlled by their actions and/or reactions. I can accept I have limits to what and where will help. I have boundaries I will not let others cross. I can acknowledge my right to improve the quality of my life by acknowledging that, "my boundaries and my limits are the real me. When I accept my limits and enforce my boundaries I am free. I am free to be Me!..,....When I let other people cross my boundaries I am ignoring my limits. My limitations are in part what sets my boundaries.......When I accept my limits I give up control. When I enforce my boundaries I give up their control of me. I am not compelled to control to keep form being controlled. As long as I enforce my boundaries I cannot be controlled. " Profile of Abuse by Dee Frances

In learning not to rescue, how not to react to their actions I stop, take a deep breath, think. Is this what I genuinely prefer to do? Is this how I want to conduct my life? Is there another way to handle this situation that would be preferable to me? Do I want to handle this situation? Is this situation my problem or someone else's? Do they really need me or will they too grow if I stay out of this and let them learn from their mistakes?

Here again is another paradox of recovery. I learn how to back off. I learn how to let others learn from their mistakes, as I proceed to do so I learn one of the most valuable lessons life has to offer me. I learn the true meaning of the term, "joy of heart." I learn how wonderful and fulfilling my life can be without feeling I have to live my life in such a way that I must continually help others to be a worthwhile person. I learn that I feel better than ever. I learn life is a true joy. I learn to wake each day being able to see with clear eyes of understanding what my blessings are. I begin to feel the joy of connecting with other people because I want to instead of feeling used by others. I learn others are more capable of handling their problems than I ever suspected. As I see they do handle some of their own problems I get more and more comfortable with the idea of not rescuing. I learn to accept how good I feel without needing to fix another to feel good about myself. I am feeling better and better about myself for yet another reason. As I let go and let others fix themselves I will also learn that much of the baggage I have been carrying around, believing it belonged to me, is not mine. When we see how much better life is, how much weight has been lifted from our shoulders, we accept with greater and greater ability on our part that this was their baggage. I was only carrying it for them. It is not, was not, mine. This now becomes a positive cycle. I have lighten my load and brighten my outlook. I have learned that many of the reasons for what I thought were my shame were not me. I can now begin to look at people when I talk. I can say with greater and greater ease the things I think. I do not fear being shamed. I know I am as good as anybody else. I need not give more than I receive to give my life meaning. I no longer feel abused and neglected. I am learning to break the behaviors I learned to survive my original dysfunctional family.

As women we had ingrained into our heads and our hearts that we as the woman would be the main nurturer of the family. We must cherish their feelings. We must put ourselves last. This is how I get to be a good wife and a good mother. How much easier could generations of men have it? To be a good wife I listen to the faithful directions of my good mother how to put myself last. Thus making it easier for the next generation of men to control the next generation of women.

As a woman whom I believe to have balanced this delicate issue of what is caring and caretaking I will say that I love my husband and family. Yes, I do without for them and sometimes they do without for me. I do for them and they do for me. At this moment my husband is washing the dishes so I can work on this book. He folds the laundry and cleans too. But this delicate balance has only come about through much hard work on both of our parts.

Here we need to define the difference between caring and caretaking. Caring is being concerned about others. Caretaking is believing that we are personally responsible for other peoples' welfare. We can fix it. They need us. They need our help. We need to help. By staying busy enough in the helping of others we give little or no thought to the main question we must answer in the process of breaking the cycle of dysfunction. The question being; Who Am I?

Up until a few years ago I would have answered that question by stating my name along with I am a wife. I am the mother of five. I like to play the piano. But sad to say none of these things answers the question, Who Am I?

Today I will answer this same question by saying, "I am Dee Frances. I am a loving person. I like to help others because I care, however in my caring I will be careful not to caretake you or anyone else. I will let you learn from your mistakes as I care about the outcome. I will help you if and when you want my help and I feel that my help will not prevent you from growing in your own direction, often from learning from an error on our own part. I enjoy helping where I can, however, I feel no need to help for the reason of elevating my own self esteem. My self esteem is in tact whether or not I help. Whether or not I can help without hindering you.

In essence you and I both need to be
what each of us seeks internally.

I can write in verse to say

what each of us would like to be.

I long to be.
I need to be.
I want to be.

Reach out to be.
Work to be.
I can be.
What I need to be.
I believe, what I need to be,
deepest longing inside of me,
IS ME!

from Poems and Growth from me to me by Dee Frances.

In my process of learning who I am and what qualities make me like others and what qualities cause me to stand out as different than others I learn that each and every human that has ever lived is totally unique. Like a snowflake. Consider this a wonderment. In the beauty of a snowfall we sometimes watch the large flakes of snow lightly drift through the air landing on our hair, our coat, our arm. Amazed that each and every snowflake is different than another. The wonder of a mind so great as to create a thing like snow. Yet snow vanishes within days. And while yet here on our earth all melts or sticks together so that to us one is indistinguishable from another. We, as humans, are also unique. Each of us have the same beauty as a snowflake. The beauty of our uniqueness. Each of us differing from another. Sociologist believe there are as many people living today as have lived in all human history. Today there is slightly over ten billion people on this earth. So in all history approximately ten billion people have existed, each one have the beauty of their own personality, their own uniqueness. We, as individuals, do not need to blend together as the millions of snowflakes of a snowfall must do to survive. Yes, in our original dysfunctional families, we may have needed to be like them, not to different from them, to survive, this however, is about today. Today I can learn to express what I want , what I need, and what I feel. I can do all these things without being selfish. Being selfish would be in effect saying, "This is what I want and I do not care what you want." Being functional is saying, "I would like to share with you what I want. When I do I also care about what you want." This is not selfish. This is functional. Being selfish would be in essence saying, "I need this and I need it at your expense." Being functional is saying, "I feel that I need this but I hope we can discuss this together, consider both of our needs and work out a solution that will work for both of us." Being selfish says, "I feel ...... and I expect my feelings to be honored by that I mean that I get my way." Being functional says, "I need to share with you how I feel about this. I will also listen to how you feel. I do not expect to always get my way, however, if you will listen to my feelings on this matter it will be easier for me to know that you care, even if the situation works out that I do not get my way." This is functional. Yet an older existing word than functional is applicable here. What is the word? Maturity.

We begin to mature as early as birth. About three months of age the baby struggles at holding a rattle. Each child is working their way through a learning process. About fifteen months of age the child begins to learn another important part of growing and maturity. The child learns the word, NO! What is also of interest is that some experts consider the mother of the child to be in a state referred to as emotional pregnancy until the child is about fifteen months of age. At this time a change takes place in the bonding between mother and child. The child is learning the power of the word no. The functional mother is delighting in the knowing that her child is growing and learning. In the case of the dysfunctional mother this can be the time when trouble begins. The mother needs for the child to follow her every command. The child begins a degree of separation from it's mother. The child is beginning to have thoughts and feelings that differ from mom. The dysfunctional mother must now do whatever it takes to keep the child in control. The child must learn not to say no to his mother. If the child does say no they will be shamed by statements like, "don't you ever say no to me." "I don't care what you want. I told you to..." in turn the child learns they have no rights and that their feelings are to be put aside for others. In this way the parent has now assured the child will be there to fill their needs, wants, and desires. The children sometime in this process learn the only way to survive is to do as told and not voice their own feelings. In the functional family the child is listened to then the parents can explain in language appropriate to the age of the child why we can or cannot do such and such a thing. When my three year old grandson says to me, "But Grandma I want to ride the horse and the car. I have my own money." I can say, "Today I do not have time. But I promise that the next time you go to the store with me and act good in the store you will get to ride the horse." His reply, "Next time I will ride the horse." Then I live up to my promise. If I tell him he has to walk and he says no. I can ask him why he doesn't want to walk. If it has been a long day and he answers as he has, "Grandma, I'm tired. I didn't get my nap today," I can reconsider it as I would a reasonable request from an adult. I do not lose my position of authority with him. I say, "Okay, you're right I didn't think of that. This time I will carry you." Or if I am exhausted myself and cannot think about carrying him I can say, "I understand how tired you are. I'm tired too. Look right over there is grandma's car. Do you think you can walk that far? Grandma is very tired. Why don't we walk to the car, drive to grandma's house and open that can of apple juice." What we are demonstrating to the child is reasonable functional living. Isn't this better than the dysfunctional model wherein when the child said no to walking to the car, the parent says something to the effect of, "I told you to walk. I'm not going to carrying you. I don't understand why you got to make a problem out of everything." It is also very likely that while this conversation is going on the child is being hit across the rump. How complicated life has been made. How unhappy everyone is.

Each dysfunctional family has it's own stressor. The stressor may be alcoholism, workaholism, drugs, hypochondria, verbal and physical abuse, death, divorce, someone's overrighteousness. Any and/or all can initiate dysfunction. Each family member does what they must do to survive. We now become outerdirected. The simplest definition of outerdirected would be to allow our self esteem or happiness to be controlled by things outside of ourselves. Thus we too become dysfunctional. If things are going good on the job, we are great. If business is slow or we lose our job it must be us. Why do these things always happen to me? What did I do wrong?

In the process of becoming outerdirected we lose our true self. We have lost our right to think different than mom. We have lost our right to peace of mind and serenity. We have lost our ability to know what is them and what is us. We have lost the pure sweet innocence of the healthy, natural child we were born to be.

Each thing we do to survive the dysfunctional system we have grown up with is called a survivor behavior. These behaviors become a habit. A habit that we keep using long after they are no longer necessary to survive. At this point survivor behaviors turn against us. In the dysfunctional family of origin we learned not to share our feelings, this was our protection. When, as adults, we start our own families we are now accustomed to not sharing with others and our spouse says, "you don't talk to me and when you do it's about some old thing at work. But you never talk about your feelings," we haven't the remotest idea what they are talking about. We say, "Of course I do, honey. I share with you more than anyone in my life." Although this may well be true the point here is, we do not share our innermost thoughts and feelings out of habit. The thing we used to protect ourselves from verbal and physical abuse has now created another family feeding off of the pain of dysfunction.

Here again we come back to the original question, who am I, do I know? We have surpressed and unexpressed our thoughts and feelings for so long that we cannot answer that question without serious soul searching. Mankind was designed to live from within himself, to fill his emotional needs. When not allowed to do so mankind attempts to fill the void, the hole in our soul, by things outside of us. In all of dysfunctional man's attempts to fill ourselves with the things outside of us they are only things. They cannot replace the hole created by ignoring what was originally there, our thoughts, our feelings, our soul.

FILLING THE HOLE

Filling the hole can also be called recovery. We have learned we are what is called dysfunctional, codependent, or shamed based. We are in the process of learning the causes of our shame allowing us to release this same shame. Our shame came about because as innocent, loving children we looked for approval from our parents. They, in their dysfunction, did not know how to show us approval. The things they did approve of us for, the things they were proud of us for, were not voiced to us out of fear of being mushy or thinking we would begin to think too much of ourselves. Thus being the case because of inaccurate understandings about self esteem. I remember an occasion when someone told me how proud my mother was of me. I replied, "Yes, she tells everyone except me."

In our approval seeking our emotional age level has frozen in our efforts to survive. We have not had the opportunity to mature through different age levels as our physical bodies grew. Adolescence will now present especially troubled times for both the child and the parent. Adolescence is the second time during the development of the child that they go through a necessary process of being different than the parents. This is vital to the emotional development of the child. The child is in a learning process. Learning about himself. What makes him tick. He needs to learn how to still love his parents without needing his parents approval for everything he does. The small child delights to run to his parents with each thing they do to show his parents what he has accomplished. The teenager says, "It's my project. I'll do it myself. No, I'm not sure I will show you when it's done or not. I'll see." The functional parent accepts this not as secretive or as a personal rejection but as a normal part of teenage growth. It is a time when the child must give serious thought to what he has been taught. He/she must give thought to the things they agree and the things to which they do not agree. What he will do the same as his parents. What he will do different. He must also prepare to leave home in the physical sense and in the emotional sense. Leaving home emotionally is not accepted by dysfunctional parents. Many dysfunctional parents expect children that have long left the nest to keep in contact with them on a daily bases. If the now adult child's schedule becomes more filled than the parent likes and the adult child cuts down on the amount of contact with the parent the dysfunctional parent takes this as a personal rejection. The child is no longer there for their every need. What can they do now? How will they be able to pull this child back to the whole of the family? The very existence of the family unit is threatened by someone venturing out on their own. In the functional family the person will be missed and cared about but his ventures will not be a threat to the family.

Dysfunction causes persons to think in all or nothing terms. When the adult child keeps in constant contact with the parent the parent receives some kind of nurturing, a feeling of importance coming from the fact their child although grown keeps in close touch. However, when this is not the case the parent expresses sentiments as follows, "all my hard work, for all those hard years, raising you was to no avail." or "Why you don't even call me. Only when you see fit to get around to it." The parent endeavors to keep the child bound to them regardless of their physical age.

The hole we are seeking to fill came about because we did not receive what is referred to as emotional strokes. I believe emotional strokes are the fuel of the soul. We were born with a healthy, normal soul. One that craved strokes both physical and emotional. If we do not receive them we continue to look for validation that we are an okay person until the happy day when someone more functional than us affirms that we are as good as anyone else. We are not perfect. We cannot be perfect. As this came about for me I coined several phrases that I still use to draw strength from as I would a boot strap. I have learned not to judge myself by the same harsh standard I was judged by by other dysfunctional people. My phrase that lightens my load in life, the one I use when I feel my actions were not up to what I would have preferred is; I can't be very, very good for very, very long. I do not use this thought as an excuse to deliberately act inappropriately. But rather I have come to accept that try as I may I will never be able to act in an appropriate way at all times. I, in my imperfectness, will continue to make mistakes. This I can accept. I have learned the true joy of not having to do things perfectly to prove to myself that I am worthy of existence. My other uplifting phrase is; I can't do everything right. I don't do everything wrong. Each of these phrases helped me to learn how to fill my void, my hole. To fill the void with what was originally there, myself. When I do, I remember that my true self, the one that was born, the real me, was not perfect. Was never going to be able to get everything right, even if she had not become dysfunctional. If I had been born into a functional family I would not have been perfect. I would however have been taught, we all make mistakes. If you spill your milk, well, let's clean it up. If you did not clean your room, then you will miss your favorite cartoons. You need to clean your room. I would have been taught that although everyone makes mistakes we take the responsibility for our mistakes. We learn from them. The thing we did was not so great. You as a person are fine. So fine in fact that I know you can grow and continue to learn better ways to handle the situations which arise in your life. I have every confidence in you and your ability. I would have been taught to express my thoughts and feelings in an appropriate way. Parents guiding and helping me through difficult situations and still allowing me to make age appropriate decisions. I would have come to know, family members are accountable to each other but they are not responsible for each other. None of these things would have made me perfect. Yes, even in functional homes people get mad. Sometimes they get out of control. How then is this different than what takes places in the dysfunctional home? If I am out of control I will at some point, stop, apologize for what I have done or said. I will say, "I'm sorry. The reason I am out of control has to do with what happened today at work," or whatever the case maybe. My children and my husband do not fear me. My children are free to come to me and say what they feel about how I acted or about what happened in my day of work. They are free to make suggestions. I will let them know I appreciate their input and their concern. I, too, know I am free to express my needs. I do not place the blame for what I just did on, "If you kids hadn't of..... I wouldn't have been out of control." These are the types of statements that caused our original confusion about what we could control and what we could not.

I fill the hole in part by knowing I am not perfect. I will never be perfect. I can work to improve my level of functionality but I will not expect perfection from myself or others. We have stopped denying the truth. We are not Alice in Wonderland. We can now stop minimizing the pain we suffered due to dysfunction.

We have come to the point that we have stopped denying the impact being raised in a dysfunctional family has had on us. We suffer from what I call chronic low grade dysfunction. Like a person who has a low grade fever but has not bothered to take his temperature all we know is we don't feel quite right. No matter what we do something is wrong. I'm sure I'm supposed to feel better than this. We cannot identify the source of our problem because we have felt this way for as long as we can remember. If we stop to take our temperature, in the literal case, we say, "It's only a low grade fever. It's nothing." This we have also done in the case of our chronic low grade dysfunction. We are now coming out of denial. The real problem was and is the styles of communication or attempted communication that were displayed for us in our family dysfunction. We will begin to fill our ever gaping hole of dysfunction when we realize that each of us has within us the ability to meet life's difficulties, to cope with setbacks as they come our way, and while doing so we are able to feel self assured in our relationships with others. Our hole of self doubt, self defeating thought patterns, has kept us believing we were not good enough, not able enough, to handle problems and face whatever painful circumstance with the strength of our own person.

The recovery process, filling the hole, does not mean we will never experience pain in our lives. It does not mean we will never overreact or feel like giving up. At one point in time my expression was, "What do I do now? What do you do when you are sick of recovery?" This was in reference to the fact that I worked a very hard recovery program. It was the joy of my life to find effective communication styles. It was joy to know that complimenting each family member on something they did well today brought joy to my heart. Hopefully it helped them but how it was helping me was that I began to notice more and more the things they did right. I was becoming more blessed by having my family members as important people in my life. But sometimes it hurt. It hurt because in a family of seven I was the only one doing it. No one said thank you to me. No one said, "Job well done." No one said, "We appreciate your efforts." One day I asked my husband what changes in me he liked. I was thinking of all my efforts in releasing control. His reply, "I like the way you quit organizing my underwear drawer." I was furious. "What? When I fold cloths I open your drawer and push them in out of apathy, lack of energy to do? Lack of caring. I have been too emotionally drained to care. All my energy has gone into letting go of control and sorting what I needed to sort. All my work and you say, 'you like the way I don't organize your underwear drawer.'" I am only human I, too, need emotional stokes. One day I said, "Why should I say thank you to you because you put your glass in the sink while you sit and watch as I clean the whole house. I think this is lop sided. Maybe I want someone to say those things to me too." Today, three years later I can delight that I did and that I do those functional things, like comment on the good things they do. Today everyone is working a good recovery program. And the three year old grandson that has been mentioned several times is the result of functional living and functional teachings. This child has had this benefit. I feel great satisfaction in knowing I can help to give to my grandchildren what I was not able to give my children. My adult children are doing a good job of breaking the cycle of dysfunction in their life's. I know with my heart and soul the role I played in setting the example even when I felt, "what do you do when you're sick of recovery?" But I got back up. Setback into negative thinking, yes. It will happen to all of us. But how did I answer my own question? I stopped, thought, do I really want to go back to how it was before I knew about recovery? I have filled my hole of dysfunction by learning that I like everyone else was born with talents, intelligence, and ability to stand up to and surmount whatever challenges or difficulties life will bring my way. As I learned to become more and more functional a phrase I used was, "The world has not changed because I did therapy. I have changed." I have learned new more effective ways to meet life's challenges.

Meeting life's challenges involve several skills. They are basically; risk taking, coping with disappointment and failure (sometimes personal failure), and problem solving. The more we fill our hole the better capable we become of carrying out each of these skills.

Recovery is learning the balance between caring about others and caring for ourselves. An integral part of caring for ourselves is taking place within us. We have started to realize the trauma we, as children, carried inside us. Carry it inside we must because no one would listen. Next we admit how we really felt about what happened to us, feel what we need to feel. I could now tell my story the way it felt when it happened. I could cry, talk through my teeth, or whatever I needed to do. I was telling my story as my hurting child felt it not as a cold rationalizing adult relating cold hard facts of this is what happened. As we begin to have the ability to let our child within speak and be heard another important aspect of healing takes place. We begin to know where we begin and they end. We are not hiding from our true feelings. I do not need to mood alter, substitute one feeling for another in an effort to feel good at all cost. When I do not need to mood alter I am giving up the role I played in my family of origin. I no longer need to fix other people and their problems to feel that I have a purpose on this earth. My self esteem is intact whether things go well or not. I have times of great joy and times of great sadness but one of the most liberating things I have learned is that sadness is not a defect in me. The fact that I have sadness does not mean I didn't get something right here. It does not mean I am not strong enough to handle the situation that is causing me to be sad. I saw John Bradshaw on a TV. special and to my joy he stated that sadness is the ability to accept reality. Sadness then is the opposite of what I had always thought. Sadness is strength to accept what is happening. I need not deny it. I need not guilt myself over my weakness when I feel sadness.

For each new definition we learn a change takes place within us that will fill another crumb of our hole, the void that was once in the pit of my stomach. The one that said, "something's wrong here."

I believe, we give to ourselves validation when we learn accurate definitions of feeling words. Our hole has developed due to our confusion.

If we cried we we labeled weak. Tears do not represent weakness. Tears represent sadness. Sadness feels like empty. For so much of my life I felt empty. I in caretaking the feelings of others would deplete all my emotional energy till I was running on empty. I said to a friend, "I have nothing left to give unless someone gives to me." I soon after learned it would have to be me who gives to me. I read an excellent example in a book by Ellen Kreidman called Light His Fire and have used this demostration myself in a class I teach called Keeping the Fire Lit. Take a picture of water add a little food coloring, red. With that we have about six glasses. The picture of water represents our energy or the love we have to give others. We pour a little into each glass. They drink it. We pour a little more. Some here. Some there, until the picture of water is empty. We think it will be filled by others pouring back a little of what they have. If this takes place fine. But we will never again have a full picture of water. How does it get full? When we go refill it. We must learn not to run on empty but to refill. Take care of each emotion as we become aware of it. If we feel sadness, cry if we need to. Talk about it with those we have found to be trustable. This is certainly better than carrying around with us the hollow feeling in our upper chest and gut that comes from a deep loss we have experienced or re-experienced.

Joy-is an overall sense of exhilaration, a feeling of lightness and a healthy sense of power. We feel spiritual. A surge of adrenalin enhances our sense of ourself and how we connect with the universe. We feel warm and good all over. Joy is a condition of the heart which has eluded those who are dysfunctional.

Joy

Joy of heart,
why couldn't I know,
why you, oh joy,
deluded me so.

Joy of heart,
few people find,
looking all around,
for answers inside.

Joy,
the reason for
my being.

Joy,
knowing a difference
I make.

Happiness,
may fading be,
but joy,
I find internally.

from Poems & Growth form me to me by Dee Frances

Anger- is a feeling of power in the gut that is followed by a surge of muscle tension in our lower, middle and our upper back and our shoulders. This is followed by a rush of adrenalin and blood flow throughout our body. This is how anger feels in it's extreme form. Many times dysfunctional people say they are not angry because they do not feel rage. But anger like any other feeling comes in all degrees. From being mildly upset to, "don't you dare touch me." This is the anger we will use to protect ourselves from a mugger, a rapist, or a wife abuser. Let us learn not to deny our anger and our right to protection.

Hurt- is a pit in the stomach. We may feel like we have been kicked in the gut, violated, betrayed or in pain. Many professional believe that hurt is anger turned inside. I, too, believe this to be true. Look back at the definition of anger. However, we in our dysfunction learned that we, a child, would be punished if we were angry with our parents. To protect ourselves from their punishing us if we had a feeling we learned to pull this feeling inside. If we shallow our power, would we not have a pit in our gut. We continue to carry this pain with us because we have not been taught how to handle negative feelings when they come up so we avoid them. The less we accept ourselves the more we ignore how bad we feel and how bad we have been treated. But our feelings keep coming back to say, "Here I am. I won't go away. I will keep coming back. Your feelings, me being one of them, are trying to help you out of this hurt you are suffering. We want to help you get this pain out of your gut. Listen to me, PLEASE!" the feeling personified above will come back. It will keep coming back until we learn what it is we need to learn to handle the negative things in our life.

Shame- at it's deepest level is felt in the lower gut and genital area. Shame produces the feeling of being broken, defective, not worthy of notice, unlovable, ugly, ignorant, stupid, dirty, awful, bad, crazy, evil and/or worthless. The bigger the shame we carry the more likely we are carrying the shame for someone else and their actions or for an entire family system from which we came.

Fear- is felt in the upper chest and breathing passages. We feel that somehow our life and our very survival are threatened. It is felt as a sense of dread and anxiety which spreads through our body unless we take actions to protect ourselves.

Loneliness- Lonely is defined by Webster as being isolated from myself. Thus the feeling of emptiness, disconnectedness, devoid of contact with fellow humans. The greater the shame we carry the greater the loneliness. Loneliness which feels as if it will eat us up. We simply want to die.

Guilt- a heavy burden that moves us to act to correct a wrong on our part. Real or imagined on our part.

Safety- feels warm, good, okay, secure, not afraid, not uncertain, connected with other people who we are assured within our hearts love us as the real self that we are finding.

Now it is time to compare what you feel with accurate definitions. Each of these new truths will be helpful in breaking down our wall of defense. Our walls went up one brick at a time. This is the same process we use to take them down. We remove one brick at a time. Each new piece of information we receive will help us to examine a section of our wall in the light of functionality, to fill our hole. In the next chapter we will discuss some of the family rules that held us within the bonds of confinement to the family dysfunction. But for now we our looking at our wall of defense. Mine began with the denial of anger, fear of anger, fear of confrontation.

I teach a class entitled Anger Handled Appropriately. When addressing how we learn not to repress our feelings I always start with anger. The first thing I do as the first session of the class starts is to ask each person to state briefly why they took the class. Always, repression of feelings is the key ingredient. Anger is the main ingredient. I believe when we come to grips with how to handle anger appropriately that we will automatically improve how we handle every other feeling we have. Most of us have been taught that anger is one of the seven deadly sins. Cain killed Abel over his anger and jealousy and the world of violence began. However, we have forgotten, "Be ye angry but sin not." As I look more into the Biblical expressions of anger I learn that anger in itself is not wrong. What I do about my anger may be wrong. Jesus himself drove thefts out of the temple in Jerusalem with whips. Was Jesus out of control? No! He was perfect. His actions were appropriate for the circumstances. These men were selling animals for sacrifice in the temple. But instead of giving the animals over for sacrifice as they had promised the purchaser, the animal stayed on their display to be sold again and again. Thievery. Not appropriate at any place but to do so in the temple was contaminating the worship of Jesus's father. His anger was appropriate to the occasion. Just as our rage would be appropriate if we were being mugged, raped, or physically violated in some way. Yes, we would have the right to fight back for our protection.

In the midst of realizing how angry I was about the effects and affects that dysfunction had on my thinking process and my life I came to know I was out of control. I did not know what to do. It was time for others to quit coming to me for all the answers. I could not even help myself. I had been trained and groomed to be tough and tough is what I was until the day where my will power would keep me running no more. I was running on empty until empty runs out. There was nothing. I could no longer avoid the pain of reality. I need help. This is a time to learn great humility. Giving up control. Giving up the idea that I can handle this. Learning the difference between willpower and self control. I had always thought they were the same. Then I learned that will power is a power that I must constantly muster up to keep this thing going. I must dig into the depths of my soul, some how, some way I must find a way to keep going.

Self control- feels good. Self control allows me to know that I can acknowledge negative thoughts and feelings. I can know I have them without preferring to have them. I now have given myself the advantage of knowing what the problem is. I need not repress this feeling because it is negative. I can pray for help. I can think this through. I can do research to find information that will help me to work my way through this negative feeling. I can talk to another, share my pain, sorrow, and confusion without feeling embarrassed. But this only came about as I learned to take the risk of talking about how I feel and felt. Not all those experiences turned out good. But the good that came from my new found ability to take emotional risk was that I learned there are trustable people and people I will not choose to confide in again. There are safe places to talk about my pain. There are people that care about my pain. I am lovable. I am loved. With this new acceptance I also learn that I have the power to change the things I can. I learn the power of letting go of the things I cannot change. Letting go of the things we cannot change is referred to as detachment. We must learn the fine art of detachment in order to fill our hole. Detaching from those that still want us to fix their problem will allow us to grow in maturity and functionality. Detaching from those that want to learn how to fix their own problems will allow both of us to grow in functional abilities. In either case detachment is the key ingredient to filling our hole, to becoming more functional. The expression goes, "detach in love." I believe that it is best to detach in love. But if it is not possible to detach in love, and with love than it is better to detach in anger and work through our anger than to stay attached and resent the person to whom we stay attached. We say we stay with them because they need our help. But realistically, can we help them if we resent them for making our life so difficult? We have believed our staying attached was keeping things in balance. Reality says, "Our staying attached enables this situation. I am contributing to keeping this painful situation going. If I detach and they choose to keep following the same course my life will be better because I am freed of the guilt I carry. I am no longer contributing to another person's drinking, drugging, sexing, over eating, under eating, gambling, working. I will live my life in the best way I know how not to contribute to any of these situations. I am learning how to let go of control. When I back off, give up control, I will feel afraid, I will worry about what will happen next, I will want to control. Now it is time to apply what I am learning. I can feel this thing and not act on it. Apply this principle to the above situation. Do not act. Let go of controlling the situation no matter how nervous you are. Wait it out. It's okay if you nervously wait it out. It's okay to be afraid. You will be afraid. After several times of this anxious, obsessive wishing I could control but didn't I began to see. This is great. That worked out fine. This didn't. But what could I have done to make it come out different. Nothing. My life is getting easier. Joy was seeping into my heart.

We are changing. We will be met with anger and rejection from those that still want us to fix their problems. We will be met with anger and rejection from those who want us to keep needing them to fill the need in them. They do not understand what is happening. They only know you are changing. You are feeling good due to your changes. They are feeling scared, "who will be there for me now?," is their fear. If we stick to our guns, risk a risk, stay detached from those who would like to pull us back into the dysfunctional system before we get strong enough to live functionally on a regular bases they too, in time, may start to see the quality of our life improving. They too may grow to want to know how to make appropriate changes. Our best way of helping them has become to help ourselves. Help ourselves to live as functionally as we can. In this way we are carrying out what is step twelve in any twelve step program. It says, "Having had a spiritual awakening as the result of these steps, we tried to carry this message to others, and to practice these principles in all our affairs." We may win them over without a word. We may win them over by their observation of how we conduct our life and how the quality of our life has improved. This is filling the hole with what was originally there, Me! My goodness of self. My spirituality. My role model for others. While doing so I do not do this for them. I do it for me. I fill my hole so that I will not run on empty. When I run on empty I have nothing to give to anyone else. If I cannot give to myself how can I give to others? When my hole has been filled I am now in the position to give to others. I can replace the part I've given away. I can do so because I have broken the family rules of denial and dysfunction.

PEDOGOGIES POISONOUS VERSES PREFERABLE

For thousands of years well meaning people have raised children under an oppressive set of rules that do not allow a child to have thoughts or feelings, actions or reactions, that are different than those they are taught to have. Most of this training has been done in an effort to teach children not to be selfish. To care about other people, and to love life, to be grateful for the things that they the parents as well as God provides for us. However, the dysfunction of the parents and inaccurate definitions of what is selfish, what is true caring about others has only perpetuated the cycle of dysfunctional thinking.

Pedagogy is a word that means we teach someone for the sole purpose of having what we teach passed on to others. We teach. That person teaches another person. They teach another. This is exactly how what Alice Miller refers to as the Poisonous Pedagogy, is still being taught to generations of young today. The good news however is; more and more accurate information is infiltrating into society today about what constitutes accurate communication and the effect and affect on children when they must stifle their feelings to survive growing up.

THE POISONOUS PEDAGOGY

1. Adults are the masters of the dependent child.
2. Adults determine in a godlike fashion what is right or wrong.
3. The child is held responsible for the anger of adult.
4. Parents must always be shielded.
5. The child's life-affirming feelings pose a threat to the parent.
6. The child's' will must be "broken" as soon as possible.
7. All this must happen at a very early age so the child "won't notice" and will not be able to expose the adults.

As my hurting child began to speak she also wrote a book called Profile of Abuse. What I refer to as the family rules came straight from my gut, not the many reference books that laid before me. They are as follows;

THE FAMILY RULES

1. We do not talk about our problems. It's private family business. But even in the family let's not talk about it.

2. We, the parents, can act any way we want. You the children have no right to say, question or think what you thin about how I act.

3. If you think my actions are bad then you are not honoring me (your parent).

4. Parents never have to say I'm sorry, you're only a kid.

5. If I do occasionally listen to your opinion and it is different than mine, you must listen and agree with me, the parent.

6. As parents we may or may not have time for you. But if we don't, no complaining.

7. You children be there when I need help, be there when I need love, be there to listen to my problems.

8. You children are the cause of my problems, I'd have it easier without you. Do you know what you cost?

9. Since you are the cause of my problems you must help fix any problems I have, or think I have.

10. We, the parent, repress our feelings. We are in total control at all times. You children must do the same. You must be in total control of your feelings. Be tough. Don't be weak and let others know how you feel.)By the way did I mention how this protects me, the parent.)

11. We, the parent, have the right to explode when we cannot tolerate how you ungrateful children behave. You children must never vent your feelings, especially anger in any way especially to us, your parents.

12. We, the parents, will seldom, show any tenderness. What do you mean you don't feel loved?

13. Do not question any or all of the rules. If you do, you prove that you a re indeed an ungrateful child.

As I began to type the family rules I remembered there are thirteen family dysfunctional rules. My Most recently released book is called The Thirteen Blessings of the Twelve Steps. I had not made the connection until moments ago that by working the twelve steps of recovery I had found what I called the thirteen sets of blessings. I have broken every rule of family dysfunction. This I knew. This is my joy. But now I have made the connection between my thirteen sets of blessings and breaking the thirteen dysfunctional family rules. Poisonous Pedagogy rules force the child to take care of the parents feelings and not their own. Throughout life we have established the pattern of fixing, minding, taking care of, what the other person feels and ignoring our feelings. If we in the innocence of our youth spoke out with, "you know what I want," we were probably told, "Well, what you want and what you get are different," or "you are a selfish little girl," or "I don't have time for such foolishness." We learned to deny our feelings as it hurt less than feeling the feeling only to be told in one form or another what we felt wasn't important. Abandonment of the child soul has now been accomplished. We are set up for problems with dependency and with relationships. If I have denied my past, how can I face the future in a functional way, with functional skills? I dare to say if we could we would not be reading the abundance of books that now fill large sections of any book store.

Herein I will attempt to share some of the differences between functional and dysfunctional families.

FUNCTIONAL FAMILIES

1. Have rules that can flex with the circumstances.
2. Take the shortcomings of the person into consideration.
3. Need not deny a problem facing an individual family member or the family as a whole.
4. Realize what they can and cannot control.
5. Detach from what they cannot control.
6. Work together as a family to do what can be done concerning family problems.

7. Offer input to family members who must work through a personal problem without feeling that person must use the information they offer.

8. Offer emotional support not guilt trips.

9. Address the thing that is going on here. Not the person as a whole.

10. State their feelings then let the other person think about it without trying to force an opinion on them.

11. Each family member knows they are accountable to each other as a family unit. I am aware that my mistakes may also hurt you. If that be the case you have a right to be hurt and angry. I will attempt to listen to your feelings and understand your reason for feeling hurt and/or betrayed.

12. Each person attempts not to jump to conclusions about any given situation. If they realize they are doing so they know the best answer is to say, "I need to talk. I don't want to think and feel what I do. Could you help me out? I'd like to know if you will share with me what is happening here."

13. Each person attempts to pull themselves up when they are down without feeling ashamed to ask for help if he/she needs.

14. Each person is free to perceive the realities of today. What is good and what is not so good about their family and their life. They needn't dwell on what was or what should be.

15. Each is free to think what they think, even if other family members do not agree they do not attempt to force their opinion on the other family member.

16. Each person is free to feel what they feel not what they have been told directly or indirectly they should feel.

17. Each is free to want or desire what they want or desire. Each is free to make choices rather than have others decide for them. From the smallest choices of what tv. show to watch, to what we wear, how we comb our hair, to what type of job training we will take. I could not be a truck driver like my father. I was a waitress like my mother. I am a writer, like my grandmother. Whatever I choose to be I must be. I have a son who is a roofer. A daughter who is a legal secretary. A daughter who is an accountant, a son who is an auto mechanic, and a son in training to be a radio disc jockey. He is a poet, a song writer, a comedian, a talker, an on the spot entertainer.

What is it that a legal secretary has in common with a disc jockey? Nothing that I can see. But they are siblings. All with different interest. All with different skills. All will make different choices. This is why the old saying, "I raised them all the same. I don't know what's wrong with so and so..." does not work. Each must be free to make choices appropriate to their personality.

The rules of the dysfunctional family are based on a master/slave relationship. The parents are deserving of respect because they are the parents. They must be obeyed at all cost. While we are not advocating disobedience to parents in love it is this domineering type of enslavement which locks in a child's silence even when being sexual abused. They have been led by the parents to believe that the parent has total control over their body because they are afterall the parent. The family dysfunctional rules set out at the start of this chapter enforce to the child that parents can scream at them but they must not scream at the parents. I do not advocate that children be given the right to scream at parents. Let the parents set and appropriate example. Let the parents act appropriate. Let's set up what I would like to call the preferable pedagogy. Instead of the poisonous pedagogy as referred to by Alice Miller that has been passed down through thousands of years of child rearing I realize that when I attempt to model appropriate behavior for what I am feeling I, by my example, am teaching my children a preferable pedagogy, ending the cycle of abuse. Carrying it on to all my future descendants. Abuse can stop here. My inner child, the natural child who hid, as well as my hurting child cried out for joy. So did my controlling child who was tired of all her hard work.

THE PREFERABLE PEDAGOGY

1. Within the family we will talk with you about whatever problems are in our life.

2. We will attempt to listen in a way to show we are trying to understand your thoughts and feelings.

3. We will seek information on how to solve our problems, personal and family problems. If we, as a family, cannot come to solutions we will seek information from

friends, libraries, doctors, or even a family therapist. Whatever is necessary to keep this family whole, loving, and caring.

4. We, the parents, will endeavor to set an appropriate example of how to handle our feelings as they arise. We will help you to learn these same skills.

5. If I as a parent do get out of control I will later acknowledge my error. I will explain to you, my child, enough of this situation without dumping adult problems on a small child, that you can be comfortable knowing that my lack of control is not your fault. It has to do with one of my shortcomings.

6. If you, my child, think my actions are bad I will attempt to allow you to express your thought to me as long as we can sit down and endeavor to talk it over in a respectful way. Respect does not mean I do all the talking. It means for you that you are trying to learn that I, your parent, make mistakes too. You express your feelings without labeling me a bad parent.

7. When I, the parent, make a mistake I will apologize to you. Your feelings count.

8. If your opinion differs from mine, we will share opinions. I will try to provide information you may not be aware of to help you learn the value of moral uprightness and caring for people. But I will do my best not to cram it at you.

9. I, your parent, will plan and schedule time for you, my child. You are important to me. If from time to time something beyond my control prevents this from happening I will explain to you why and we will reschedule our plans. I will make sure that it does not become the rule that other things take over my plans with you.

10. I, the parent, will make sure not to burden a child with adult problems.

11. Regardless of how expensive things are today I will not conduct myself in a way that conveys that I regret supporting my children in a financial way.

12. I will take care of my feelings as I become aware of them. I will do my best to role model appropriate ways to handle each feeling. I will not think you are arrogant when you feel good about an accomplishment.

13. I want you my child to ask questions about anything you do not understand. Because I am secure with my own feelings I will not be intimidated by your speaking up about any aspect of your life. I will feel honored and respect that you trust to share your innermost thoughts and feelings with me, your parent.

The family dysfunctional rules set us up to deny our right to know and to understand what we feel as well as why we feel it. The most sacred of all rules is not to question the rules. We learned denial. We minimized not only our dysfunction but the problems it has brought in our present day life. To keep the Poisonous pedagogy intact comes another set of rules . Dysfunctional families believe;

1. The duty you feel toward me is love.
2. Parents know best.
3. Be nice no matter what.
4. Adults deserve respect, children don't.
5. To be good you must obey without question.
6 You're so arrogant, don't you dare think too much of yourself.
7. Touching is not necessary in this family.
8. Act thankful. No matter what you think.
9. Be nice again, no matter how awful it feels.
10. We're right, we're the parents. Aren't we? Our power reigns supreme.

FUNCTIONAL PARENTS SAY

1. If you feel duty towards me I am glad you have a form of responsibility. I prefer to have your love.
2. Parents don't always know best. I've heard tell, "out of the mouths of babes."
3. I think you have many nice qualities. But remember no one can be nice all the time.
4. As your parent I feel I deserve respect. I also know children deserve respect too. Respecting you means I listen to you. Try to understand why you feel as you do even when it is different than how I feel. Especially if it is different than how I feel. If I don't understand I will pray to a power higher than myself and ask for help.
5. To be good means you attempt to work with me in a spirit of cooperation. This is best done if you understand the reasons for our rule. Feel free to ask.
6. Feeling good about a personal accomplish is what will give you the power to know that you can change things about yourself that you do not like. This does not equal

arrogance.

7. I love to touch and hug you. Will you hug me too?

8. I am attempting to teach you, my child, how to show thankfulness and gratitude. I also don't like false shows of thankfulness.

9. We can attempt to speak to each other in a respectful tone and at the same time convey that we are upset with each other. This I allow as your parent. But not everywhere or everyone in the world will allow this. If you feel that a certain person or place is not a safe place to express your feelings you need only hold them in until you come home. Here at home you are safe to say what you need to say. I only ask that you attempt not to vent them on me. I will allow you to express them to me.

This too is a part of the preferable pedagogy. This I believe comes under the part that says, "I care about you. I will attempt to listen and to understand how you feel."

We are learning how to break the cycle of dysfunction. The preferable pedagogy is the set of keys we use to do this. We use it for ourselves. We use it for our children. This is functional living. Not perfect living. Notice the rules say, "I will attempt to..." "I will do my best to..." But when we are living by this standard of dignity we have ridded ourselves of shame. Shame and dignity are the exact opposite. According to Webster's New World Dictionary shame is - a painful feeling of having lost the respect of others, the loss of honor. On the other hand dignity is- the quality of being worthy, a position that deserves respect. This position worth respect is called THE PREFERABLE PEDAGOGY.

It is preferable to denying and repressing. Preferable to years of pain and suffering with which we cannot connect a cause. Preferable to the alcoholism, drugs, sexing, overworking, overeating, undereating, or gambling that many dysfunctional people have used in the attempt to fill the ever present void that lingers in the pit of our stomach. Lingering and controlling our soul. Yes, our soul is in the pit of our stomach. It got there by swallowing our thoughts and feelings. Swallowing the lump in our throats when we felt different than we had been told to feel, knowing it was not safe to express that thought or feeling. Roget's International Thesaurus describes our thoughts and feelings as our soul.

In order to break the power of the dysfunctional family rules we must break down the power of should thinking. Should thinking is a negative thought pattern that keeps implying that somehow we never quite meet up to standard. What standard. Who's standard? In the dysfunctional family each family member is controlled by the should thinking expressed in the following;

1. Each family member must think on how it should be because the present is not bearable. If we could make it like it should be we would be okay.

2. Who sets standards of what each of us should be. We tell ourselves what we should think, what we should feel. This is a demonstration that what we do feel is guilt. Guilt for not feeling what we should feel. Feeling different than we were told.

3. We fear our feelings are bad they are not what we have been told to feel under similar circumstances.

4. Each person feels guilty when they want something different what what we've been told to want. Many of us were told it was wrong to want anything. "What you want and what you need is different." Of course not everything we want is a need. But it is a human need to have some things just because we want them. If this is not the case we are existing not living.

5. Each person must role play. He must accept the role he accepted at a very early age without the knowledge of the impact it would have on the rest of his life. Sometimes we are forced into a role at birth that has been determined by parents before our birth. Case in point. A young single mother who has never felt loved or wanted. Now she has her own baby. This baby will be her love. He is special. She will always be there for him and he will always be there for her. He can fill the needs she would usually have filled by a spouse. This process is called spousizing. The child is now expected to fill the needs of a husband. He will work to do so with all his might. Little does he know this role was cast for him before his birth.

The family rules have prevented the open expression of feelings. Repression of feelings is probably the biggest cause of death.

Ulcers kill. High blood pressure kills. Heart attacks and strokes kill.

Alcoholism kills.

Drugs kill.

Over eating kills.

Undereating kills
Overworking kills.

All are methods used to mood alter. Substituting something that makes us feel good because we cannot talk about what is hurting us. What is hurting us is the inability to talk about how we feel and know that others do care to listen. Others do care to understand. Others do care about us.

The denying of our emotions has brought us to this state of dysfunction. Brought us to a time when our body's coping mechanism will copy no more. It is time to learn why the repression of feelings has hurt us and how to make appropriate changes in what we do with our feelings.

Emotions are defined as strong feelings by Webster's New World Dictionary. These feelings are so strong that they are put into motion as our basic powers of protection. Emotions are signals from our body that tell us of a need or a loss. Energy is generated from our emotions allowing us to act effectively to take care of ourselves in the circumstances we are presented. As we learn to understand our feelings (our soul) we understand how to have a healthy relationship with another. Emotions are prime to our state of physical and mental health. Emotions are direct expressions of our thoughts. Our thoughts translate our experience giving us important information about what we need to do , what we want or how we want and/or need to change. We have the ability to express all emotions at all intensity levels. Each emotion ranges from the very mild to the very violent. We can feel conflicting emotions at the same time about the same subject. This is referred to as ambivalence.

When we are functional we have the ability to sort through feelings of ambivalence. Ambivalence only befuddles dysfunction. Living with a rageaholic causes us to feel that we must repress our anger. We repress our anger as we are literally not capable of dealing with their anger and our anger. We must deny our own anger. We should not be angry. Maybe they cannot help it. We deny our right to anger because of their anger. We are in effect denying our right to protection from their anger. Dr. Robert H. Curtis tells us in Mind and Mood, that anger and fear are essential for an individual to survive in a life-threatening situation. Anger is our strength. Without anger we are their doormat. We deserve whatever they dish out to us.

Rage is the ultimate end of the anger spectrum. This occurs when someone or something is trying to stop an action we want to pursue. They are attempting to control us. We attempt to control back in our efforts to keep from being control. Their rage at not being able to control us is met with our rage at not being able to control their attempts to control us.

We are learning to break the cycle of dysfunction. This chapter has set before us some of the differences between functional and dysfunctional families. In learning how to improve our level of functionality we must learn the art of detachment and how we will be affected by what is called both the Forgiveness Process as well as the Grieving process. Two different names for the same thing.

DENIAL VERSES DETACHMENT

In my process of recovery one of the hardest things for me to feel like I was getting this straight was to know the difference between denial and detachment. In regards to a very painful issue I thought I was doing a great job of detachment only to find through a mistake that would cost me half of the then manuscript, Profile of Abuse, that I had only denied. I have since come to know that if I feel, I am fine. If I feel nothing, if I feel that regardless of the tragedy going on with other people I love and how it will effect the relationship between them and I that I am a okay than I have come to know this to be a state of denial.

In my process of learning the art of attachment I came to realize some situations will go on for years. Our only source of sanity will be bringing ourselves back to step one, realizing I have no control over other people. Then step two, knowing that a power greater than myself can and will give me sanity if I take step three, turn it over to him. Dysfunction taught us to deny the reality of how bad this situation was/is or how badly we hurt. Functionality is teaching us to face our pain. Look at the negative in this circumstance. Face and/or discover how we feel about the negatives. Cry. Talk. Write. Rid ourselves of as much of the negativities as our body will allow. Draw strength from knowing we are able to handle even the very painful. Even if we feel we have been carried by our God we can draw strength from knowing we are capable and he was wanting and willing to help us through this most difficult of problems. Now look for some positives. If nothing else we can be positive about our new abilities. When I was nervous about doing things in the past I felt like, "I can't do this." This I would always say as I went about doing whatever I perceived needed to be done to cope with the situation now present in my life. Soon I would come to the conclusion; "I'm doing it. I'm doing it nervously, but I'm doing it." This would bring me to another conclusion: "Strong means I do what I have to do to handle the circumstances of my life. I can cry while I do it if I want to." All of these will not become some of our positives. All of which will allow us the confidence to know we need not deny. We can however detach. One of my positives in any situation is always: I do have the right and the ability to detach. Detachment does not mean we have to quit loving them. As I expressed to someone I love, "I love you. I love you no matter what you do. I also have pain when I see you...... I realize it is your choice how you live you life. But because I love you I will continue to hope and pray that you decide to change some of your choices. I love you no matter what but I have decided it is not best for either of us for me to act like everything is okay. I cannot associate with you as long as these are your choices. But in my heart I love you. If you decide you want help I will be there for you. Just let me know."

This is not the help of rescuing and denial. This is helping if and when they are ready to acknowledge their need for help. If I am trying to help them when they see no need for help, I am denying their denial. I must now come out of denial about their denial. This is the process of detachment.

I do not have to intellectualize my way through my problems. I believe that as the imperfect humans that we are we will for the real of our life suddenly find a series of things has built up on us when we thought we were facing our feelings as they come up. This I believe is due to the fact we do our best as part of being functional to face our feelings as soon as we are aware of them. The key here is the statement, "as soon as we are aware." Our bodies have many emotions at any given time. We consciously cannot sort and separate them all. Our subconscious stores the rest until they build to let us aware they are indeed there.

We have come to know how we benefit by detachment from situations we cannot control. Detachment means I do not let their emotions control my emotions. I know what I feel and why I feel it.

As hard as it may be to detach I believe it is easier to detach from those who continually disapprove then it is to stay attached to those same dysfunctional, disapproving persons. I believe attachment to dysfunctional persons hurts more than detachment. If that were not the case why would any of us be reading recovery based information.

In each of our processes of finding out for ourselves what is denial and what is detachment, when we resort to our old habits of denial and when we are best at applying detachment we must be aware of the differences between the two. Listed below are qualities of each;

DENIAL

1. Denial must shut off this pain. I must not think about it. Different from taking a break from thinking about it. Realizing that I can give it a rest and come back to it when I'm not so emotionally exhausted.

2. Denial attempts to forget this happened or

3. Denial says, "Yes, it happened but it was no big deal. It had little or no effect on me.

4. Denial takes the blame for how others will..... I am denying they are responsible for their actions.

5. Denial causes a chain of events that will worsen the situation until one day it hits us like a bolt of lightening.

6. Denial says; "Just because I don't talk about it doesn't mean I don't know about it."

7. Denial says; "Did I see what I thought I saw? There must be a reasonable explanation."

8. Denial is an effort to disavow any consequence of our actions or the other parties actions.

While this chapter is entitled Denial verses Detachment we cannot discuss this subject matter without discusses forgiveness. Most of what I know to have been denial in my life was due to my misperceptions about forgiveness. I wanted then and now to be a forgiving person. I thought, "Why bring it up? Forget it. I can surely forgive this." As I faced my issues, as I learned to know I must detach to be able to forgive, I came to ponder, detachment or denial which, I thought it was forgiveness. Nope wrong again. Anytime I find myself saying, "I'm not really upset with them." "I don't hold it against them." Anytime I find myself saying these things over and over again, or talking about the same situations over and over again, I have not forgiven, I do have a grudge. I say them as part of rationalizing away my negative feelings. "I don't have a problem here. The problem is......" Maybe it is. However, I also have a problem. My problem: I am trying to deny how I feel about...... Rest assured that when we keep talking about a situation our bodies and our mind is trying to say to us, "This does bother you. Let's get some help. Let's talk about it hoping someone will validate our feelings. Let's talk about it again." Our body is trying to be our own best friend. It is telling us to take care of ourself. "Get this thing settled. Quit denying." When we have detached to sufficient enough degree to have peace of mind because of our detachment, we need not keep discussing it. We thought we had detached but using the above information we can think about it and decide if we truly detached or if we had denied, AGAIN!

DETACHMENT

1. Detachment feels the pain of the present situation long enough to decide what will be best for us in this situation.

2. Detachment is a deliberate knowing the results that may come my way due to my letting go of this situation, positive and negative. I can detach knowing I may lose a friendship or someone dear to me and still detach knowing it is the most positive action I can take in my life. I know this is for my betterment.

3. Detachment is aware of but does not take the blame for other people's responses to my detachment. When I detach I consider the needs of the other people involved. I know one of the healthiest way I can be of assistance to them is to set a healthy example of functional living. I can have true peace of mind in the hope that one day they too will want to copy the example I have set.

4. Detachment makes my life freer and happier. My decision does not come back to haunt me.

5. Detachment is aware of the impact of these circumstances.

6. Detachment is the ability to accept the things I cannot change, the courage to change the things I can, and the wisdom to know the difference.

7. Detachment has made a choice to remove ourselves from a situation or person knowing we will benefit from our choice. It does not mean we will not hurt because of it. I think it means we we hurt less. Our pain in the detachment process is a temporary thing. We may from time to time have pain because we miss this person. We can grieve our losses. This pain, however, is not the continuum of pain which exist with attachment.

Are we coming to know the differences between denial and detachment? We will learn more about the difference every time we discover we have denied where we thought we had detached? Another opportunity for learning has presented itself to us.

DETACHMENT AND FORGIVENESS

Dysfunction is the epithemy of staying attached to people who use us to fill their internal needs. Needs that would be healthier filled from inside theirselves. They are dependent people and we have become dependent on them. They, however, cannot meet their own emotional needs. We cannot expect them to fulfill our emotional needs. It now becomes time to learn how we go about filling our own needs. When we fill our own emotional needs we can never be abandoned. When I place my emotional needs in the hands of another I always risk my needs not being fulfilled. I can guarantee this need will not be fulfilled. One of my basic human needs is the ability to think and feel and make decisions for myself. Taking responsibility for the outcome, for good or for bad.

Dysfunction causes us to become dependent on people we don't like or love. We do not like them but we need them. We need their approval. We begin to hate and resent them. We tell ourselves that having someone is better than having no one. We stay in abusive relationships for the most illogical of logic. We are more afraid of change than we are of the current abuse. I have come to learn that the only thing we have to fear is fear itself. Change can be frightening. Change is also enlightening. The changes I made during the course of my therapy and subsequently by living a functional life have brought me to the writing of several books. I always wanted to write. Write I do. Without the changes that I made in my thinking process I would never have begun my writing career. This is a passion for me. Two of my main fields of interest were writing and psychology. Writing helps me to stay functional and I have the joy of knowing that some of the things I have to say have made the difference in the lives of others. While at the same time I do not need to do this for my self esteem to remain intact. Self esteem I have. Writing I love. I have learned that I need not keep things the same to be safe. I need not fear change. Change represents growth. Positive changes allow me to know that my work has been worth my efforts and reinforce to me my abilities to change the things I feel I need to change. Negative changes help remind me that I am not perfect. I only attempt to balance my life while knowing that I did and do have setbacks. I strive for balance without reaching for perfectionism. I understand that; Balance is perfect. We're not! .

I know that when I repress my feelings in order to stay attached I will feel, hurt, fear, anxiety, and fear of confrontation. When I take care of myself by detaching from responsibility for other peoples reaction I feel love, joy, and enthusiasm. I will also feel respected, understanding towards others, caring about others as well as myself, I will feel that I am being treated fairly and desire to treat others fairly. I have learned to take the pain that life has given me and use it to learn. I use the things I learned in dysfunction to remind me how much dysfunction hurts. When I feel I do not have the strength to detach. I recall how much dysfunction hurts and how different and liberated my life is today. My dysfunction had left me with the ability to diagram a sentence and with little communication skills. Today I possess the most precious of all possessions. I know how to communicate in any type of circumstance. I can handle difficult people. My self esteem is intact.

I have learned that balance means I am able to accept a compliment while also being able to listen to and accept a suggestion for improvement. Each of these abilities allows me in my own special way to be able to detach from those very dysfunctional who would prefer to keep me needing their approval thus validating to them that they too are important.

This is referred to as being undependent. A well rounded individual. We carry ourselves with dignity. We live our lives from a position worthy of respect. We have a natural need for other people in our life. I remember Proverbs says those who isolate themselves will fair badly. To need to feel a connectedness to other people is a natural feeling and need. If we ignore the need to connect with our innermost self and put connecting to other people as more important then we will continually be frustrated and disappointed. Remember the word lonely means to be isolated from ourselves.

We are working on being self respecting, self reliant, and self sufficient. We are not working on being stiff necked, cocky, or inflexible. All words used by Roget's International Thesaurus as meaning the same as self reliant. Just as pride can be used to denote a false pride, a system of covering up our own mistakes out of fear of embarrassment, or a healthy sense of pride in our personal accomplishments without using our accomplishments to feel we are better than others.

The process of becoming undependent requires us to develop the ability to detach. We are freeing ourselves from dependency, entrapment, enmeshment, codependency, and dysfunction. We are allowing ourselves to start the process of working toward our personal goals. When we are caught up in the fury of their dysfunction and their need for our help we are what is called enmeshed. Wrapped together with them. Their problems become our problems. Plus we must deal with our problems. In the midst of this is it now even reasonable for us to feel that we can set personal goals and have the ability to reach them. Detach. Detach from their need for us. Give to ourselves the ability to reach out for our own goals. Give to them the opportunity to grow by learning how to handle their own life.

If I detach from others I grow as a person. I can be me. I can know why I feel as I do. If I am attached to them their feelings trigger or even control my feelings. My detachment process is established when I set and enforce by boundaries. When I enforce my right to be such and such, do such and such, or feel such and such, I am in effect saying, "Here I am, I would prefer to agree to disagree, but if you are not able to agree to disagree and still respect another even though they are different than you, I must detach. For my own self respect I cannot let your feelings dictate my feelings, my thoughts, or my actions. I will act in a way to consider your feelings but I need not be controlled by your feelings.

When we were enmeshed, the opposite of detachment, we told ourselves this is what good people do. They need our help. They don't know how to.... We worked over time to help them. Then we began to resent them. Resent the very one we are endeavoring to help. What we are really attempting to do is to prove to ourselves that we are capable of the very things that our parents always told us we were not capable of doing. At the same time we can prove it to others. We can move in with a fix and they will see the power and the ability I have. As much as we come to resent them is the extent they come to resent ourselves. We are always there with a fix. Never do we give them credit for being able to figure something out for themselves. Never do we give them credit for having strength enough to work on their own problem. Isn't this what we resent mom and dad for? Now we have done to others what we hated someone doing to us. Thus the cycle of dysfunction continues.

How do we break this cycle? We break the cycle by learning how to detach. Detach even when we are nervous. Even when we are sure it will not work. What have we got to lose? Our current way of doing things has only brought us frustration, disappointment, rejection, resentment, their rage, our rage, the constant feeling of being used. Try something new. DETACH!

Becoming undependent is being able to take care of ourselves without guilt. Guilt for not helping them. Guilt for detaching. Yes, you will probably feel guilty for detaching. I can only suggest not to give in to these feelings of guilt. Remember; old habits die hard. After a while you too will find joy, contentment, satisfaction, and a new life are yours. You will also proclaim to others; It was hard work but worth every bit of effort I put into it. And it is.

We will probably recall how scared we were. How we did not think this will work. That is why it is called a leap of faith. It is a leap of faith because we let go of controlling habits we have used all of our lives to reach out for something we are not sure will work. But work it did. We were scared and now are delighted to know that being scared only confirmed how normal we really are and always were.

As we learn to detach we are able to press on. We can now see how things in our past are affecting our life now. It is not over and done. The actual event may be over but done it is not until we come to understand how that thing that happened to us affects our feelings about things today. With our new understanding comes freedom from fear. I did not understand why I did not like recliners. Why I could not cut my hair without feeling uneasy and why I felt so bad when my husband said he loved me. When he said to me, "I love you." I would say, "If you knew some of the things I think you wouldn't." Sometimes I would say, "I'm not what you think I am. I'm only trying to be what you think I am."

One of the greatest blessings that has come my way through recovery is; **to be able to sit all the way back in a recliner chair, to cut my hair without feeling dirty, and to know that when my husband says, "I love you." that I am worthy of his love.** Now when he says I love you I am able to smile, take a deep breath, and let the goodness of his love spread throughout my being. I do not think him nuts for loving me. All this has come about by learning how to detach from negative events and negative people. I seldom have to deal with the word distress. Stress is produced by trying to handle too many emotions at one time. We eliminate much of our stress by being honest with ourselves. Not by denial or repression of our true feelings, the ones felt by our inner child or true self. The child we once were. That small but hurting child can come to visit me and I will listen. I listen not with ears of fears. I listen knowing her pain. Knowing what she has to say is important. Also knowing most everything of importance I have learned from her. My hurting child, my painful emotions, let me know when and where I need to detach to protect my own integrity. This is our chance to be different.

The tie that binds us to the dysfunctional family is broken as we stop seeking approval by staying attached to a system that has not worked out to the benefit of any of it's family members. We have gained through our detachment approval. That's what we have been looking for our whole life long. Approval of the real me. I can be confident that I will be there for others. I will be there because it is the earnest desire of my heart. Not because I must to attempt to fill a need in me, a need in you. Dysfunctional needs that never were filled by my fixing or by their needing me to fix. We will detach when we decide we are sick of the pain and turmoil of dysfunctional life.

Of the most important of all judgements we make in our life none will be as important as the judgment we pass on ourself. How we judge ourself will be the core of our universe. It will affect everything we think and believe in our lifetime and how we connect with everything else in the universe.

To honor ourself means we become willing to know what we think, what we feel, what we want and need, the things we desire, what things cause us suffering, what frightens us, what angers us. We need to feel what we feel. If we don't we are but a shell living out the life term of this body. Here we are speaking of our soul, our total self. Roget's International Thesaurus equates soul with our thoughts and feelings.

What I know best about denial is it is not detachment. With detachment we are learning the art of caring about ourselves. We are learning that to honor ourselves is not selfish. We must honor ourselves before we can truly honor anyone else. We are beginning to connect our present pain with past dysfunction. At this time our learning process will include a positive judgment of ourselves. This can better be referred to as the forgiveness process. We can forgive ourselves for the wrongs we have done knowing we can make amends by living our lives in such a way that we do not perpetuate those same wrongs. We take a honest look at ourselves and change the things we see that need changing. Perhaps we too were an abuser. If I now live my life in an non-abusive way I demonstrate to those who may have been hurt by my actions that my state of heart is; **if I could do this or that over I would do this different. If it was within my power to do so I would. But I can promise you that from this day forth I have changed that particular aspect of myself.**

This I believe is the next best thing to being able to do it over. We cannot go back in time but we can learn. We can be thankful that time does not stand still only for all parties involved to be stuck in pain for the rest of their lives. We can overcome thinking of ourselves as stupid, incompetent, untalented, and hating the way we look by admitting how we honestly feel. We are no longer in hiding from our pain, our hurting child has now found the joy of being able to speak. We have come to befriend our hurting child. She is not a mere figure of speak. She will come out alive and kicking proclaiming her right to be heard. Her right to cry tears of pain and sorrow. And her right to ask of our real self sincere and honest forgiveness. When she started to talk we were in effect dredging up the past. We are not chopping off our weeds at ground level. This time we ware pulling them up by the roots and throwing them away. I am learning to take responsibility for my part in any given situation. This angried me a great deal in the beginning. I felt they did this stuff, not I. My Part! You're kidding, aren't you? But what exactly was my part?

I allowed the size of my body to become a self esteem issue. For years as an adult I allowed myself 500 or less calories a day to maintain a hard earned figure. I did not know the danger of some of my practices until I read in the newspaper about a famous musician who had died from eating disorders. This sacred me. I did not share with others what I had been doing. I did change the dangerous habits. Of course, I began to gain back my weight.

I became a fixer to prove my self worth. I was the one everyone counted on to hold everything together. I could list more but what has been listed is sufficient to see that how I had responded to the original circumstances was due to my choices. Now I must make another choice. This choice was not only about change. This choice was about forgiveness of my inappropriate choices and learning to increase my degree of function. Now I must learn how to forgive myself and others so I could stop the dysfunction of the past from ruining my future.

The forgiveness process includes five steps. They are:

1. DENIAL , first we deny. Many, I would venture to say will stay stuck in denial for the entirety of their lives. We numb ourselves in order not to feel the pain. The problem becomes that along with numbing comes no pleasurable feelings of love and generosity. To this I balked. Of course I feel. But now that I have worked my way out of and through dysfunction I know the difference in the intensity of my feelings of love, joy, kindness, goodness, mildness, faith, long suffering, and self control. I do unequivocally state that what I felt in my dysfunctional days were mild feelings of love and the whole gambit of human emotions. Dysfunction is about repressed feelings. Feelings we have tried to kill. We felt it was unsafe to have them. Our very existence depended on their death. And as I listed the range of human good emotions just a few sentences above I realize what they are from. Maybe you recognize them too. Why not check out Gal 5; 21-22. These are the fruitages of God's spirit. These then are the results, fruitage, of having God's spirit work with us. Coming out of denial will put us into touch with each and every one of those feelings. We no longer need to use compulsive disorders such as alcoholism, drug addiction, sexaholism, food addictions, workaholism, inappropriate behavior such as laughing when we want to cry, and crying when we are angry. No wonder we felt crazy. Releasing the craziness is granting our right to peace of mind. But the first step is to come out of denial.

2. Anger- as we start to accept our denial system and understand the realities of what happened to us we will be angry. We can no longer deny our losses. One of our biggest losses will be our childhoods. Recently I went to see The Lion King. This story is the perfect illustration of how the lies and manipulations of others in our childhood

causes us to lose our childhood. If you have not as yet seen it, I suggest doing so. If you have think back on what happens to the young lion cub immediately after the death of his father. Think too of how he felt when he learned the truth and the actions he proceeded to take.

This story is the perfect illustration of child abuse. The child was lied to and manipulated. He grew up entirely different than he would have. When he finds out the truth he is an adult. At that time he proceeds to take actions to rectify his life situation and that of his family. He did so in his anger.

I was much like the lion cub. My anger flared for all to see. I did not care about their reasons. I did not care about their feelings. I only cared that I had been manipulated and used and I had fallen for it. I became like the main charter in another children's story. That of Humpty Dumpty. I came crashing down from my wall. Crashing down from my position of control and power. The anger of a lifetime rushed in on me. Not only for the things of the past but for the present. Their anger of the present that I was talking. My anger of the present that I felt like Humpty Dumpty, I fell into pieces and it was only I who could pick up the pieces. I being overwhelmed by new circumstances and the lack of control had zero confidence that I would ever be able to fit the pieces together again.

3. Bargaining- Now has come the time to bargain. Bargain my way out of my anger. I can save face. Mostly I can save face with myself. I do not have to have this loss. I can gain what I need to gain and not lose what I was in fear of losing. I can gain my personal confidence and still hold onto my family and earn their approval. This is the farthest thing from the truth. But each and every one of us in our grieving process will attempt to hang on to what we fear we will loss and what we hope to gain. Our losses may well be other persons. Persons we love. It is at this point in time we learn about detachment. Strangely enough the beginning of the detachment process may start with the other parties. We have been hanging on, doing for them, trying to help them, giving all our energy to them, only to find they are the ones that say, "Leave." "Get out." "I don't need this." As we become aware that all of our efforts are only appreciated when things have gone their way we may well move backward into anger. Anger that

we have been used. Angry that we let them. As the realities of my anger struck me one after another I moved into the next stage of the grieving process, that of depression. This is not mere sadness. This is out and out depression. The difference between sadness and depression is; sadness is the ability to accept the negative things that are happening in reality. I accept those negative aspects of my life knowing that although I hurt I will work my way through this sad period of time in my life and continue to have my personal strength to continue coping with my life positive and negative.

4. Depression- however is my lack of ability to cope effectively with negative events of my life. I have trained myself to turn negative events into, what did I do wrong? The true trademark of depression. Our depression is a direct result of our bargain not working. We're sick of it. Grief and severe mourning set in. Isn't this what denial was about? Isn't this what we so wisely planned to avoid? Didn't we know it would come our way? Yes, we did. We knew in our soul that we must not dare to be different. We must not grieve what the family sees as okay. My depression now takes me back to anger. When I came to realize this is called the forgiveness process I was furious. I screamed! I yelled! I cried! I wrote, FOR WHAT! TO FORGIVE THOSE WHO WILL NOT FORGIVE ME. FORGIVE ME FOR WHAT? MENTIONING IT!

I now would waver back and forth between all of these stages and my anger. All my life I had striven to be what I thought was a forgiving person. Now I am presented with what is the true and most accurate way to forgive and I was angry. Again it was time to look at myself. Never mind whether they see a need for forgiveness. This has become about me not them. This is about what I allow myself to hang on to and what I am willing to release. This is about how I can accomplish peace of mind. Here at last I have the whole ugly picture. What do I do now? Am I really the type of person I had credited myself with being? This is indeed a question worth the asking. To continue my progress in recovery I must do more than release my past pains inflicted by what others did. I must also accept that I carried those pains with me wherever I went. I believed some of them. I used those things to my disadvantage. Because I believed some of the assertations that were thrown my way I was the one who had low self esteem. I am the one that wants to feel better. I am the one who wants to offer my family better. If they wanted recovery, they also would be here. They are not. I must now come out of denial about their denial. I now reach the point of

5. Acceptance. I accept I cannot do a thing about them. I would prefer they too work recovery. I can also accept that one day they might but in the meantime I will not hold my breath waiting for you. This is my life. I accept the wisdom of the serenity prayer. In my own words I say,

God grant me to
learn from the things I cannot change
give me courage to change what I can
give to me wisdom to understand and work with the difference.

Acceptance means I let go of control. I quit trying to get the other guy to see my side. I need to see my side. I can forgive myself and learn the true joy of forgiveness and with it the joy of heart that approval of myself will bring.

Acceptance does not mean we are happy about the situation. It does mean we have given to ourselves the ability to accept reality whether or not it is favorable to us. Certain memories will hurt. A happy stage is not acceptance. Acceptance is knowing our struggle is over. We can now be aware of where our own negative thoughts and feelings came from and not allow them to control our present day conduct. We have gained the ability to live with our situation realizing the beauty of the serenity prayer, the ultimate form of detachment. We emotionally detach from dysfunctional others. It is a loss, sometimes a great one. Whether our loss is great or small we are prepared to live with our losses in order to retain our gains.

We needed to feel anger and great rage. We needed to blame. We needed to rid our bodies of the negative events of the past. We had to endeavor to bargain. We had to cry. Cry our heart out. Cry out the feelings that would find no words. Our hurting child has finally gotten our attention. It now became time to hold her, caress her, and tell her how much I have always cared. When she healed, I, too, healed.

No one can tell us how much time our grieving process will require. I did not want to be controlled by what others had to say about the amount of time spent in my grieving process. I will grieve what I need to grieve. I will let go when I am ready to let go. I heal at my own rate and in my own way. I am putting into effect what I am learning about how to be the true me.

ACKNOWLEDGING THE BENEFITS OF NEGATIVE FEELINGS

Dysfunction and/or abuse has caused us to be fearful of our feelings. Fearful of anything negative. Fearful of our joys. Dare we to be happy when others are hurting. Dare we laugh at something they do not consider funny. We only know we fear fear. How can we in our struggles to be functional learn to accept fear?

Anger had been our enemy for many years. Up to this point of this book we have discussed some of the benefits of acknowledging our anger and how it can work out to our good. The same principle is true with each negative feeling. Had we grown up in a functional home we would also have learned this during our childhood.

Fear does mean to be afraid. Emotions are our body energy sending to our mind what we need to know to handle any given situation. Healthy fear protects us from harm while not incapacitating us. Fear of fire for example. Fear gives us wisdom and discernment. We sense fear where we could possibly be hurt. This is to our benefit. Our childhood days have taught us well how to detect dangerous situations. We can now become functional and still keep the ability to know when we are in danger. We are learning there are safe and unsafe places and people to share with. If we sense this place is not safe we will feel fear. Pay attention to your feeling. Healing from dysfunction is about paying attention to what we know to be true. Fear now becomes our protection. We need not quake with fear. We need only to acknowledge our fear and take whatever actions may be appropriate for our own protection. Maybe, all we need to do is to leave the present situation. This is not the fear of denial. Not the fear of confrontation. This fear produces wisdom as to what is in our best interest for our protection.

We are now past the point of fear. We dread a person or a situation. Dread is worse than fear itself. We can now easily be so overwhelmed with fear that we are immobilized. Pushing us through the depths of fear and into anxiety. Emrika Padus and the editors of Prevention magazine of 1986 compiled The Complete Guide to Your Emotions and Your Health therein suggesting Cognitive therapy to build skill in handling difficult situations. Our relapses will be fewer and shorter and less intense as we build confidence in our new ability. We can also learn to use humor as a coping mechanism. Laughter triggers the brain to release catecholamine, a hormone which causes the release of endorphins, the body's natural painkillers. Helping us to confront even dreadful situations. A person with a good sense of humor can use humor in different stages to their advantage.

1. to ridicule their own shortcomings. We can cry as much as we laugh but either way the end result is the production of endorphins to sooth our nerves.

2. We can laugh at the hostile behavior of others.

A person with a good sense of humor can handle a wide range of problems without giving up as easily and bouncing back to try again at a faster rate. We can eliminate our association with negative people, detach. Add joy and laughter not gloom and doom to our lives.

How to Master Your Nerves written by Peter J Steincrohn M.D. and David J LaFia M.D. states, "systoms of today may be full-grown plants of yesterdays seeds." Pertaining to dread we can understand that the thing we dread today is rooted in the things that have happened to us somewhere in the past. We can greatly lessen our anxiety associated with such as we learn how to set and uphold effective boundaries, more will be discussed about boundaries in a later chapter.

Anxiety could best be described as a condition that leaves us physically and emotionally helpless. We become exhausted by always having to be on guard. Systoms of anxiety are sweating, pounding heart, cold clammy hands, dry mouth, dizziness, light headedness, numbness and/or tingling of the hands, feet and other body parts, upset stomach, hot or cold spells, frequent need to urinate, diarrhea, discomfort in the pit of the stomach or a lump in the throat. Any of these systoms can come on suddenly or gradually over minutes or hours. Systoms can last seconds, hours, or days. Situational anxiety is brought on by being put into a situation that triggers a dangerous situation of the past . The way we think can contribute to or relieve anxiety. Dysfunction has fostered negative thinking patterns. If we now dread a situation believing we do not have the ability to protect ourselves or our loved ones anxiety mounts. Our only protection is to begin to change how we think. Mobilize ourselves. We may go about avoiding situations that cause us to feel dread or anxiety.

Now we have less ability than previously to confront what we dread. Our dysfunction is allowing us to deny it's reality by avoiding issues we do not like or feel we cannot handle. When anxiety is interfering with how we are able to conduct our life it is time to get help. There are several things I can learn to do when I begin to feel anxious. They are:

1. Breathe slow and shallow. In and out very slow. I will feel bad but this will pass. By taking the time to force myself to breathe slow and shallow I am making myself stop from overreacting to the thing I dread. This may be merely seeing someone I had a confrontation with or fear I will have a confrontation with. They walk into the room and my heart starts to pound as I dread their walking my way. Breathe slow and shallow. I am forcing my mind to relax by allowing more oxygen to flow through the brain. If I hyperventilate, I actually worsened the condition. The less oxygen the brain receives the less my body is able to focus on what I need to do. I become dizzy from lack of oxygen, which is also a sign of an anxiety attack. My body gets the cue to rush head long into an anxiety attack.

2. Okay I feel tense. I can tense all my muscles as much as I possibly can, then relax, tense, relax. Slowly. I am starting to feel more relaxed.

3. I can think of the worst situation possible. This is the one that helps me the most. When I start to become fearful, I think-what is the worst thing that could happen here. Think of an end result. Realize I've handled worse than that. I begin to relax. In the case of the person I dread walking toward me I say, "Worse thing that can happen here is they and I argue." or "They walk past me in order to snub me." "Okay not so bad. I've been snubbed before. I lived through it."

4. Tell myself, "I will not run. I will not run." This was hard for me. I ran out of meetings where functional parent -child relationships were being discussed. Why? Anxiety, fear, pain, and anger. I felt I had applied those suggestions but it sure did not work out for me. But as I learned one night to sit in my seat. I hurt. I shook. I cried. But I stayed in my seat. I learned that I need not run. The conversation in this

religious meeting will not kill me. The intensity of my anxiety although I felt like dying did not kill me. I learned not to run. Not to run.

5. As the intensity of our anxiety builds say, "I still will not run. I still will not run."

6. Think about something pleasant. Relieve some of the stress.

7. Realize, "I am really scared but I will feel better. Everything is temporary."

8. I will feel like this will never end. Tell myself, "Everything ends. Then I will feel better."

But I think the most helpful thing was a phrase commonly used in recovery, feel the fear and do it anyway. I can know I am fearful of this. I can know I dread this. I can grow. My anxiety can become less and less frequent with less and less intensity. All to my advantage. I am learning that I am a capable person. I have come through some pretty rough stuff. I did not always know how to handle it. Therefore I ran, I avoided, I feared confrontation. I also sought help. I learned better more constructive ways to handle life, my feelings, my shortcomings, and my fears. Each of which have brought about me. The me of today. The me that is competent and confident. The me that craves to share with others some of the things that have helped me through denial, fear, anxiety attacks, and low self esteem. I can state all of the above with no shame.

Shame too can be used to our advantage. Shame lets us know we are human and limited. Shame tells us we need help. If it had not been for the shame I carried I never would have sought therapy. I never would have become the person I am today. I like the person I am today. I have been all to look at and use the things I have experienced to become better not bitter.

CONSIDERING OTHER FEELINGS

We have considered anger, fear and dread, and shame. Anger can be our protector. Fear can teach us discernment. Dread and shame can make us aware we need help. Sadness we've learned is the strength to accept reality. Guilt is our conscience former. I am aware the thing I did was not so great. I am okay. I am okay because I want to improve. I want to learn about myself.

Basic human powers are to perceive, to know, think, emote, feel, remember, and imagine. These are all skills we will be required to use throughout our life. In dysfunctional families we fear the truth. Our inner self has been whispering in our ear, "all is not right here." We know internally this is dysfunctional. We dread knowing the truth in a conscious way. We learn how to substitute feel. I like best how I phrased it in Profile of Abuse, I quote,

"We laugh to cover sadness. Look how happy I am. We cry when we feel anger. We must not be angry. Our substitute feelings become habits. We look for sex when we want love. We eat to find comfort when we want a hug. We reach for a drink to escape our reality, enter compulsive behaviors, all in an effort to escape (deny), escape from how we honestly feel."

When we deny our emotions or cover them up with what is a more acceptable emotion we deny our life energy. We substitute feel for so many years we are now totally unaware of what we do. Compulsive disorders become the only way we can feel what we would have normally felt before substitute feeling. Our dysfunctional background has left us emotionally battered. Battered and bruised. Bruised and confused. We do not know the difference between happy or sad. Nor do we know the difference between tears and weakness. We do not understand the true meaning of being helpful. Our definition of being helpful is to forsake everything we want and need to do something for someone else that we neither have the time or the money for. This is not helpful. This is the definition of a martyr. We do not know the difference between sickest and anger. We say, "They make me sick." when we mean, "I am angry." Is it any wonder that life seems to have passed us by or that we have trouble communicating with others. We say, "We're out of milk." When what we need to say is, "Do you have the time to go get some milk?" Is it any wonder we are confused? Sometimes we are literally sick from the frustration and stress caused by all the confusion. The stress we feel causes the muscles of the stomach and small intestine to spasm. Hydrochloric acid rushes to the stomach. The combination of muscle spasms and stomach acid eats away the lining of the stomach resulting in an ulcer.

Guilt too has turned against us. Healthy guilt allows us to feel badly when we have acted wrongly. Because of our dysfunctional background we do not know the difference between healthy guilt and shame. Honest guilt begins to feel like shame. We have not learned how to share our feelings. Our feelings remain pent up inside. We never receive the satisfaction of feeling honest guilt, going to someone we trust, telling them what happened, and learning that probably everybody has done such and such at some time or another. We never get the validation of knowing we are normal. Honest guilt pent up turns against us as we feel, "If they knew this they would not think so much of me." Honest guilt has now turned into shame and depression. "I can not get this right," syndrome.

Our imagination is stifled as we have not been trained to look for new possibilities. Without new possibilities we have no hope for a brighter day.

Love is the most important emotion. Love can mean many different things. We, dysfunctional people, are looking for unconditional love. The type of love we never received as a child. The dramatics are that if this unconditional love is not fulfilled in childhood we will keep searching until the day we find it. Many don't. Many find their way into therapy and recovery. We now learn the love of self that is not selfish. Not arrogant. Not denying the rights and feelings of others. The love that cares about others and is able to balance my love of other people with love of myself. Taking good enough care of myself that I will be able to help others, when I want, when they want, without feeling that I must to be a good person. This helping is giving me connectedness with other people and the joy of being a cheerful giver. This I believe is what Jesus meant when he said, "love others as you do yourself."

Desire is an impulse to obtain. To look for pleasure, to long for something. I longed for functionality. How about you?

Hope is when we feel the future is uncertain but we think it could be better. The reason I hope is.....

Determination is our ability to keep up the good work when all else and everyone else seems to be against us. Determination is our most positive emotion. It is our most effective tool to work for change. Determination gave to us hope. Hope reinforced our determination. Determination gives us a reason to look for adequate accurate information about how to go about changing for the better.

As we go back into the sections of this book that consider different emotions and how they effect and affect us, stop to meditate over each one. Think of how it's definition applies to you. How did your dysfunction revolve around the mislabeling of your emotions? I was told I was mad when I was having anxiety attacks. Throughout therapy I talked about anger. Almost a year into therapy I said in essence that I was so angry that I might as well be drunk as my head was on the other side of the room anyway. At that time the therapist turned the discussion into one about anxiety. From there I went to the library. Dysfunctional people mislabel, misidentify, most emotions. This is why it is called dys-function.

Our repressed feelings equal our dysfunction. Our emotional withdrawal. As we learn to express appropriate emotions we are able to adapt to whatever the circumstances of this day, this minute, or this hour. We are learning how to accept change. We are learning how to let go with greater ease. We have had losses. We have come to accept our losses. Our acceptance does not mean we have to like them. Then we free to say, "This loss really hurts. But I know I am learning and growing. I detach with greater ease." And maybe one day you will find the same kind of joy when I heard these words come out of my mouth about a given situation in regards to detachment, "am I doing this because it is easier?" The minute I said it I knew how far I had come. Detachment had actually gotten easier than attachment. My feelings were becoming more appropriate to the situation. I expressed them with greater ease and less tears, with time and practice. The working of an honest recovery program is the key ingredient. I can do this for no one but me. I do this for myself. Others are free to join me. In this I delight. Every time we demonstrate a positive action to another "we are in effect inviting them to come along for the most wonderful journey we will experience in all our life. It is a journey of excitement and adventure. It is full of risk and losses. But better yet it is a journey that will be worth every ounce of work we put into it....It is a thrill to know with all confidence I can do this. I am doing it. I will keep doing it. .....I will have times that I fall, times I won't feel like it is worth the effort, but all of the above invalidate themselves as I begin to think how much better my life is since a few kind, loving people offered to me a positive thought, or maybe two, and invited me to take a journey down the road of life, not existence." from Positive Thinking Easier Than you Think by Dee Frances.

What do you think? Shall we consider our other feelings? Will it be worth the effort? Can you really become functional?

In answer I can only say, thousands have. Thousands more are joining us in our travels down the road of recovery. How about you? I can guarantee you will be met with love, honesty, and truth. Your thoughts and feelings will be listened to. Others who have been where you are at today do know, do care.

TEARS

It seems to me that the general population of the world takes great pride in, "I don't cry." My three year old grandson has a whopper of a black eye. When I asked him how he did it he told me he hit his eye on the side of a metal swimming pool at a picnic. Then drawing back his shoulders with pride he said, "I didn't cry."

I said, "Did it hurt?"

"I didn't cry grandma."

"I know you just told me that but what I want to know is , did it hurt?"

"Yes, but I didn't cry."

"Is it okay to cry?"

"Yes."

"So it can hurt and you can cry if you want to?"

"I know grandma but I didn't."

Even the smallest of children seem to take pride in not shedding a tear even when they have never been shamed for crying. This three year old though has a ten month old brother who not only is a constant crier but a constant screamer. So added on to this conversation was,

"Joseph cries all the time. He's a baby. I'm not."

"Oh, I see. But you have seen grandma cry."

"Yes."

"Is grandma a baby?"

"No."

"So we can cry if we want to?"

"Yes, but I didn't want to."

Tears are a natural mechanism for adapting to our emotional stress. A way of equalizing sadness, anger, surprise, fear, or frustration. Sometimes fear represents joy. Have you ever been so happily excited that tears run down your face? Tears produce endorphins. Endorphins are a hormone the body uses to sooth our nerves. If the body feels it is getting overwhelmed even with joy the natural release of tension is accomplished through tears.

At the Ramsey Clinic Dry Eye and Tear Research Center in St. Paul, Minn..... Dr William H. Frey II has studied the biochemistry of emotional tears. The results of his studies show that gender is the biggest determining factor in how often a person cries.

Boys and girls up to about age twelve cry with the same frequency. After age twelve girls cry more frequently. Totaling about four times the amount as their male counterpart.

Frey believes that the male gender has a biological bases for crying less than females. Culture of course has much to do with whether or not it is acceptable to cry. Some of the standard rules connected with not crying are;

1. If you cry at work make sure your boss doesn't see you.
2. If you're a woman don't cry in front of a man.
3. If you're a man don't cry in front of a woman.
4. If you're a man don't cry in front of another man.
5. Best yet whether you are a man or a woman don't cry at all.

If a man is not supposed to cry in front of a woman or in front of a man that leaves him sneaking off by himself to weep when he needs. Hoping no one will notice. No will will find out. Cultural stigmas definitely influence and control how often we allow ourselves to shed our needed tears.

Physical reasons are involved in the fact that women cry an average of 5.3 times per month whereas a man cries 1.4 times per month. 85% of women said they feel better after crying while only 73% of men confess to feeling better after a cry. Could this too be due to cultural influences of what a man should be? He should be strong enough not to cry. A real man should be able to handle this. All doubts planted by our culture.

71% of men report only watery eyes and women (47%) reported flowing tears. Six percent of women said they never cry while 45% of men reported never crying.

An interesting physical reason associated with women crying more than men is that emotional tears contain a hormone called prolactin. This hormone is responsible in aiding milk production and is released in response to stress in both genders. By age 18 females have 60% more prolactin in their blood than men.

If we have come from dysfunction that taught us not to cry, to be tough at all cost, that tears were weakness, think now of what we have been deprived of. An emotional release for both genders. In addition for females the lack of a healthy cry on the average of once a week may even inhibit us from nursing our new born infant. Nursing has proved to be a great aid to emotional bonding between mother and child. So before our next generation of three year olds is taught by us or learns through observation, "it is best not to cry," that generation is also being affected by the lack of our tears.

I feel that I can best sum up the value of tears by including the following poem. Let's not allow our past dysfunction and repressed feelings to continue by being ashamed of tears. I can gladly say there are times when tears flow down my face freely and I don't care who sees them. I am not weak. I know my own strengths and if a few tears flowing down my face and off my chin will release overwhelmed feelings of either sadness or joy, lightening the stress within me, allowing me to get up and say, "I feel better now. What is it I need to do to handle this situation?" So be it! I care not what another thinks. This is my detachment from worrying about how others judge my personality. If another who sees my tears thinks I'm weak this is something they themselves must work out. And maybe one day they will also find the joy of tears. For this I pray. However, in the meantime, I will not stifle my tears to accommodate their dysfunction.

Tears

Tears, I was forbidden.
Tears, are weakness I was told.
Tears, are for fools and those weak of heart.
Tears, inward swallowed, engulfed me.

Tears, hidden from the world.
Tears, I seldom shed.
Tears, a sign of weakness,
is the thought that ran through my head.

Tears, I can express.
Tears, release tension from my mind.
Tears, can be of joyful things or
Tears, to grieve the things I lost or never had.

Tears, taught me of things I need to know.
Tears, released memories of old.
Tears, released the hurting part of me.
I'll cry no more internally.

Tears, have added to my life.
Released my soul from inner strife.
Tears, aided me in my search.
Tears, help the body function in a healthy way.
I now not need to tear no more for thoughts of yesterday.

from IN THE MID OF NIGHT by Dee Frances

ANGER PAST AND PRESENT.

The grieving process states first denial then anger. Although I knew not about the grieving process I followed every step. Coming to learn about the grieving process helped me to see that although I was intensely angry I am a normal human. I didn't know any of this. But after reading it I wrote; ALL THIS AND I'M NORMAL!

So out of denial I was. Now I am angry. Angry about the past. Angry about the present. What do I do now? I can't stand to feel like this. This doesn't feel so good. This is what denial was all about, not feeling this.

I was angry about how I had been treated. I was angry that I accepted the guilt for other peoples' actions by feeling that I was dirty. I was beginning to understand the rules of dysfunction, the DON'T CRY SYNDROME and how it had affected me. In the previous chapter we discussed a few of the values of tears. All of which we, the dysfunctional, were denied. I had held in my tears for so many years that I can honestly say that during my childhood years I was in a constant state of sadness. Now it was time to be mad. The expression goes, better mad than sad. Although it did not feel that way to me. I felt struck. How awful I felt. Okay I know I have a right to be mad. Okay I know anybody would be. Okay. But this feels like it will never end. But end it did.

Our anger is, was, or will be over never having been validated. Never finding the unconditional love for which our sweet innocent child was looking. Maybe never being held. Never being told we did a good job. Never being allowed to know that we are important to this family. Never feeling that it makes a difference that we are here.

Yes, I knew I was needed. But I thought I was needed for the things I did. I wanted to help my mother. I wanted to make her hard life easier. I also wanted to be loved just because I am. I was so caught up in doing to help others in the family that my fear was, "what if I stop doing for them? Will they still love me? In fact, do they love me now? Maybe they only care because they need my help?" Being complimented as being the good kid didn't help my plight. I was now stuck in the role of the family heroin.

When I was told I was good, I thought, "If you knew some of the things I think and feel you wouldn't say that." Not being able to accept their compliment added to my guilt. Now it was time to be angry. Angry at their dysfunction. Angry at mine. Angry at their betrayal. Angry at myself that I , too, had learned how to betray myself. I must now learn how to forgive myself for not knowing how to care for my internal needs.

I came to read in A TIME TO HEAL written by Timmen Cermak that I could not bust forth out of my anger. I needed to work my way through my anger. The preposition makes all the difference. I could not bust out I must work out the roots of my dysfunction, like it or not I must face it, stay out of denial about the realities of childhood family life.

The family unit is the base of society. Many debates have been cast over the cause of the fall of the so called Holy Roman Empire, included in those debates has always been the disintegration of the family structure. Home has been declared throughout history to be a haven from the outside world. But for the dysfunctional and/or abusive family this is not the case. Children find reasons to be out in the world rather than being at home. Children immerse themselves in school, in sports, or in fun rather than face the dreaded idea of being at home.

The family structure builds what we are and how we connect or disconnect with the rest of the world. The family needs what each individual needs. Each of us need to feel worthy. The family as a whole has this same need. If the family is shame based, family secrets must be protected at all cost, the family as a unit feels the shame cast over their heads and throughout any type of structure of family they may try to build. Each person has a need for intimate relationships. So does the family. If this family is the outcast of the neighborhood each family member feels resentment for themselves as a person as well as the family as a whole. "What's wrong with my family?" "How dare they shun our family."

We all need to be needed. We need stimulation and a reason for being. Our reason is to know we connect with other people and the universe. Our reason is to know with firmness of heart that it makes a difference we are here. We are loved. We feel loved. We are affirmed.

The family needs parents that have a healthy relationship. Ones who are secure enough to parent their children without feeling intimidated by their children. Not parents who depend on children to fulfill their own emotional needs.

I was a problem solver. I felt responsible for everyone. I was afraid of my feelings. I felt guilty for many of my feelings. Feelings I would come to know were normal human feelings. Feelings of ambivalence. Feelings of love and hate for the same people. Guilt and confusion fed the process of more guilt and more confusion.

Now I am angry. Angry at others for controlling me. Angry at myself for letting them. Angry about family lies. Angry I was deprived of a childhood. Angry at being used. Angry that I needed them so badly. How is it I could need someone I resented so much?

Dysfunction has made the parents unavailable to the children's emotional needs. The parents are so consumed by how they will survive this situation or that that they completely ignore the needs of the child. They are engrossed in the details of survival, this is what I must do not to keep everything going.

The parents being unavailable to the children now creates a vacuum. Nature abhors a vacuum. Nature sucks everything into the vacuum trying to fill the inner void. The father will now spousize a daughter. She can now fill many of the needs he wishes his wife would fill. Another child will act as a parent while dad is away becoming super responsible, or as everyone says, "very mature for his years." Someone else relieves the tension in the home by becoming the family clown. Another brings honor to mom and dad by being a straight A- student. Another the scapegoat. If there is trouble, who will find it? "I will," says the scapegoat or rebel. Parents now can become more intimate over their concern for the child. The children have accomplished what the roles set out to do. HOLD THIS FAMILY TOGETHER. Thus children learn they can control. Children perceive they have control over other people. This sets up dysfunction in their minds and controlling actions become habits. These habits, or control, will only be broken if at some point in time they become open to learn more effective ways to handle the situations that arise in their life.

No one has taken the role by choice. If the relationship of the parents is not functional the players line up to fulfill their part as if players in a game of chess. The roles have been set. There will now be no fluctuation within the family. This is the part you play. Each player locks into their role to feel needed, to feel connected. The battle lines have been drawn and the battle of survival within the dysfunctional family continues until any individual within the family attempts to break free from the family dysfunction.

Any family member, probably most family members, will take on multiple roles. No matter what else is required of you to survive here you cannot give up the original role. Is it any wonder that as we start to take it knowledge of what is functional that we feel anger griping us, holding on, not wanting to let go. The process of letting go is what will one degree at a time free us from our past dysfunction, however, I felt it was not me holding on to anger. It was anger holding on to me. I wanted free from it's grip. I wanted to get on with my life. But my anger taught me it did indeed have it's hold or control on me. I could not ignore it. The personification of anger was holding me, daring me to face it. "Come through me not around me. I won't let you. This time you cannot avoid confrontation. Face the thing you fear. FACE ME! I will not let go of you till you take a long hard look at my face. See what you need to see. Never forget it. Use me to your advantage. I will see you again from time to time but you will never be afraid of me again. You will never see this intensity of me again. I am your lifetime of anger and frustration. But I am willing to become your friend. Look at me and I will start to release my grip."

Anger about family lies, alcoholism, drug abuse, parenthood, whatever the case may be are all justifiable. If children were told, "I only took a shallow to calm my nerves," as they saw mom or dad pour a bottle down the sink, children resent then deny the reality of what they saw. "They said they only took a shallow." If the wine was really for chicken with wine sauce why pour it down the sink? Why not take your shallow and then make the wine sauce? Life does not make sense. Shame basing deepens as children sense things are being covered up. I must now give my family dignity. I did not know I could not give my family dignity. I can only give dignity to myself. My family has to find their own.

I need to feel my own feelings. I don't need permission. I will not ask permission. It is a loss. I can no longer deny the unpleasant. I have looked Mr. Anger in the face and said, "Yes, I know you." I looked long and hard. I know his presence but do not fear it.

We need to deal in order to heal. We have led our life by being Mr. or Mrs. Fixit We don't want to hurt anyone. I won't hurt anyone. Not only will I not hurt anyone, I can help you no matter who hurts you. We need to fix to know no one will suffer as I did. Emotional pain is emotional pain. Pain that turns physical. Finding it's way through all our body members. We seek release. Even short lived release is release. Enter compulsive disorders. Now I feel better.

Finding a better way will involve digging into ourselves, finding out how we felt when the original events happened and how we feel now. I believe our feelings are not our personality. Every personality has every feeling. I believe what makes me is what I decide to do with my feelings. A person who wants to stay in the grip of anger is of a different type than those who want anger to release them. Both types will however need to embarrass it before they can release it.

My anger is not a sin. Ephesians:4:26 "Be ye angry, and sin not." K.J. Translation into modern English would be, 'Know you are angry. But don't use your anger to do what you know to be wrong." I can trust myself to handle my anger appropriately. I need not run. I need not attack. I only need to relax. By acknowledging my anger or any other negative emotion I can allow myself to see;

1. where I need to change.
2. Where I need to set a boundary.
3. where I need to detach
4. when I need to call for help from my God.
5. When I need to learn more about what is going on with me. What else is gong on here besides what is going on here? Is this situation similar to past events where I was hurt? Do these people act like other people I find difficult to get along with?

By considering these things I learn about myself. If I become aware of the need for change than my negative emotion has served me to my benefit. I can change any negative thing about myself. I can change the things about myself of which I do not like. I am now in the process of resolving my inner conflicts. Inner conflicts produce anger. If I face my anger, resolve inner conflicts less anger will be created in the future. All to my improved quality of life.

If a child is told a parent is sick or tired when they are drunk the child knows something is wrong (the feeling). The child's mind really doesn't want to know mom or dad is drunk (the thought). Now comes the conflict. The child is uncertain, anxious, shame based, and dysfunctional.

To resolve our inner conflicts we must acknowledge them. This helps us to understand what happened. The formerly buried conflict is now understood and we feel better, freer, and happier.

It would be a good idea to seek professional help if:

1. we feel totally overwhelmed.
2. do not feel others would understand our plight or our feelings.
3. have felt as in number 2 for most of our life.
4. Realize we overwork, overeat, oversleep, drink alcohol, or take drugs to be able to carry on with our life.

Seek help! Do it now! We cannot handle it all. We all have limits. We are in step one, which says, "came to know we are powerless." We are out of solutions. Professional help can teach us how to establish healthy limits, personal goals, and healthy boundaries. We can now learn to be considerate of our feelings, and still be considerate of the other person's feelings. I did not know both were possible. But in my anger I learned to say, "Enough!" "Enough, this is what I need and it is about time someone listened to me. All my life I put your needs before mine. Now I want you to listen. If you cannot I'll have to reconsider my position in this relationship." If I want others to take me seriously when I say, "Listen to me." I must first set the example by listening to myself. I need to quit shutting out my needs.

When I say, I want, I need, I feel I am mature enough to know I will not get everything I want, I need, or I feel. I would however like to know you care to listen to what I want, I need, or I feel. I then will do my best to listen to you say I want, I need, I feel. Now we are in a position to work a compromise where each of us gets part of what we want. A compromise is not me giving in and you totally getting your way or vice versa. A genuine compromise is when all cards are put on the table. Everyone gets to say what they really want. Then each is willing to flex. A resolution comes about when it is decided to do part of what each person wants or this time we'll do it your way but tomorrow I want to.... Okay it's agreed upon. Everyone's feelings are validated. Everyone is taken into consideration. True communication is being established. We forfeit much anger as we are learning we are cared for while others are learning effective ways to show their caring. They are learning because we are demonstrating to them how it is done by releasing anger. Saying I want, I need, or I feel. Not pulling it inside of us then feeling resentment and anger toward them. We are learning the healthy alternative.

Share our feelings. Most of all share our anger. Know others can know we are angry, they will not leave. They can know we are angry and forgive. They can know we are angry and love us anyway. We can learn the beauty of being loved despite our faults. We learn we can goof up and be loved anyway. I believe if we learn how to share our anger and know we are safe, know we will not use our anger to hurt others, we will also begin to share all our other feelings. This is how it worked for me. I began to tell my husband my anger over things in my life. Things I never shared before. He did not think me terrible as I thought he would. I had to take the risk. What I gained was unwavering confidence in his true love. I shared my anger. Soon I could say, "Do you know what I'd like to do?" or "Stop, no, I need you to listen. It is not good enough for you to hold me while I cry then we go do it your way." This I now considered to be tender, caring, invalidation. Soon he too came to see how invalidating this was. He made appropriate changes. I love him all the more for doing so. But this change came about because I was angry enough to say, "This is what I see gong on here. I need you to listen to my needs." I had to get angry before I could express those needs. Through anger I learned he is adaptable. I now do not need to let it become anger. Through anger I learned proper expression of my feelings. I grew. He grew. We grew as a couple.

Weak boundaries are the biggest factor why we cannot tell others how we feel. We let their feelings control or dictate our feelings. We now become angry that no one acknowledged our feelings. When we learn we can express our feelings of anger and still be loved and have approval we also learn we do not have to be perfect or play a role to get approval. We are learning to stop seeking approval.

If a sharing person is not present, write it down. It could become a book.

Our constant struggle with anger is due primary from not being taught how to deal with anger. We observe how others deal with anger. They act on their anger. We observe people getting hurt. We get hurt. We don't want to do that. We believe nice people control their anger. Yes, they do. Nice people learn appropriate ways to express anger but this we do not know. What we learn is, "do not explode." So I must, "Hold it in." Neither of which is an appropriate solution. We hold it in, hold it in, hold it in, until the muscles and nerves of our body cannot hold one more thing, then we explode. "oh, no," we tell ourselves. "I blew it.' We acted just like they acted. We have proved to ourselves anger equals violence. Now we must try again. Hold it in. Hold it in. Hold it in some more. And the viscous cycle repeats itself ingraining deeper in our should thinking that anger equals violence.

Try a new solution. Don't hold it in. Don't vent it. We need only express it. I believe the difference between aggressive and assertive can be summed up in the following definitions;

aggressive - to vent our feelings on others

assertive - to express our feelings to others.

Again it is the preposition that makes the difference.

Conflict is a fact of life. True it is not a desirable fact of life. It is however a fact of life. When I say I am no longer afraid of anger it does not mean I desire to have it. Realistically I have come to know that no matter how hard I work to keep things nice there will be times I will be angry with others. Times they will be angry at me, times we will be angry with each other. Conflict is not a sign of abuse.

Healthy families conflict. While they do not desire to conflict they are also aware that it will happen from time to time. When it does functional persons are not afraid other family members will think less of them. They are aware the other persons may not like what they did but functional persons will not label them as ignorant, bad, stupid, or a jerk because they disagree. Even when they disagree strongly.

Repressed feelings turn into other feelings. When living in an atmosphere of fear or constant anger handled inappropriately, children are afraid. Repressed fear turns into anger. Anger that is in effect saying, "why do we have to live like this, all I want is for all of us to show love for each other."

Children in their fear, learn to work overtime to please those they fear, for their own protection. Or they rebel in their efforts to draw attention to the family needs, "We need help. Will someone please help us?"

Children in their efforts to please learn how to avoid anger. Their avoidance of anger has now dysfunctioned their ability to handle conflict. Results;

1. They run from conflict.
2. They learn to keep things nice at all cost so no one will be hurt due to anger.
3. They become obviously angry to insure their protection.

In each solution above the child has learned control. "If I can keep things nice no one will be hurt." Thus we learn to take responsibility for other people's actions. If someone said to us, "You're not responsible for what they do." our reply would probably be, "Of course not. I can't change anyone but me." But what goes on at the conscious level is quit different than the subconscious level. Keeping things nice amounts to saying, "If they do this, I can still do this. I can make sure things run smooth so no one gets hurt." Our attempt at control no matter how good the motive is an effort to control how others act. We will be resented for it. We then suffer more, as we feel, "I helped them and look how they treat me. They don't appreciate what I do." We must let go of control. As we do we will have less anger.

When children rebel in their anger they too are saying, "If I can draw enough attention to this family I can see to it they get help." They too are taking responsibility for the problems of the whole family. Will they be able to handle anger appropriately? NO! They have learned to be aggressive. They have learned to let their rage show, to control, to make sure no one gets close enough to hurt. And their obvious rage has brought results. They too have learned control. Their method is the opposite of the, "keep it nice at all costers." Theirs is, "I can stop you. I can make sure things are within my power. Watch and see what I can do." Their anger is their control.

Anger handled inappropriately is control.

Expressing anger or any other feeling appropriately is called functional. This is what we lack. Expressing our emotions is communication. The parents dysfunction now reinforces the poisonous pedagogy. What the parents feel is what counts. They are right all cost. The cost is the happiness of everyone in the family.

In the functional family what everyone feels counts. Regardless of their age.

To overcome our fear of anger we must learn to realize;

1. where we have had mistaken ideas about anger. Ex. anger equals violence.
2. feel our anger. Justifiable anger is just that justifiable.
3. let ourselves remember the thoughts associated with our anger.
4. Look at the thinking process we have that is associated with our feelings of anger.
5. make a reasonable decision if we choose to act on our anger. Ask God to let us know what to do. Ask the person with whom we are angry. They may give us what we need. They may not. If not we must handle our feelings the best we can.
6. Don't be controlled by our anger. Detach. Detachment does not mean we don't care.
7. Discuss our feelings as appropriate. Do not talk to a drunk. Do not attempt to hold back someone who is walking out the door. Do not try to explain when someone is screaming.
8. Take responsibility for our anger. Do not scream or name call. Eliminate the phrases, "You make me angry." "Look what you did to me." or anything similar. Instead say, "When you..... I got angry." or "I'm very angry. I don't want to be. We need to talk."
9. Talk to people we trust. Have our feelings validated. This is best not to be a put down session to the other guy. This is an attempt to explain to someone we know can keep a confidence if we require that, what our feelings are. This is to help us to understand others care about us. It is not for the purpose of degrading others.
10. Work off anger energy. Hoe the garden. Walk. Clean.
11. Don't beat ourselves or others for feeling angry. Walk away. Don't get physical.
12. Write letters we don't intend to send or keep a journal. Write it out. Work it out. Sometimes I can still work out my anger easier on a word processor easier than with another angry person. If it still is necessary to talk to that person we will be more

effective. In writing I learn what my bottom line is. I can now go to them and say, "I need to talk. Something that is upsetting me is...." I can go straight to the point. I have greatly increased the probably of them listening to me. I am cool enough not to name call or degrade their person because I don't like something they did.

13. Deal with guilt. Separate baggage. This was them. This was me. They did. I felt. Yes I had a right to feel as I did. Guilt is greatly lessened even gone.

In coming to grips with our feelings we must look back into our childhood. We will be angry. Angry that those who claimed love for us would now be angry that we want to heal. Step thirteen comes to play here. Sort guilt. The insults they threw our way to keep us in control no longer work. We have learned to separate baggage. At the very least we are angry enough to say, "Not this time." If the other person is an alcoholic or other compulsive person they cannot see the needs of others. The spouse is so wrapped up in what they need to do to appease the alcoholic that the children are ignored. We cannot be children we must be at least adult enough to care for ourselves. We are also caring to the parents. We cannot play. We learn other survival tools. I used reading to escape. When I was in fifth grade my teacher said that the neatest thing about books is that you can do anything from within the pages of a book even travel to distant parts of the world. That turned me on. I could go anywhere or do anything.

A book called, "Little Miss Perfect." talks about how children adapt to the family system. Children often become short little adults, No one notices how much they are hurting. Children who find it necessary to adopt adult-like coping personalities still LOOK AND FEEL like children. They still have childish emotions, childish impulses, dreams, and childish fears. This hit home with me[1]. No wonder we hurt so badly. It reminded me of something else I read. Fifteen years ago I was reading an article that spoke about depression in children. It also discussed signs of depression. The article mentioned that if any of these signs persisted for more than two weeks parents should seek help. I started to cry. What moved me so? I had felt those things most of my childhood and my parents did not notice. I cried out loud, "two weeks, a lousy two weeks what about a whole childhood. Where were they? How could they not notice something was wrong?"

I now must notice what is wrong. I can acknowledge the inner voice that talks to me. It is the true me, the natural child. She is telling me what I really want, need, and feel. When my controlling child would say to me, "you are selfish," my real self would achingly cry out and say, "I'm tired of doing without." "Why should I do without." By the time I tuned twenty four I starting doing little things for me. It got easier and easier. I can buy a dress, go to a movie, or buy jewelry, whatever with no guilt at all. I have come to realize that I am as important as anybody. I am not arrogant because I like many things about myself. I respect myself. I love myself. I can play without guilt. I am freeing myself of anger and guilt and learning to be what I need to be.

BEING DEPRIVED, BEING GRATEFUL, BEING ME

I wrote these following pages in early 1991 but I have decided to insert them here almost as I wrote them then.

My father used to buy a bag of candy and pass it around to all the kids in the congregation. I'd watch. He never gave me any. Then one day I said, "dad can I have some?' His reply, "No, this is for the kids in the congregation." I never asked again. I felt he cared more about them then me.

Candy wasn't the only thing of which we were deprived. We had holes in our shoes and tattered cloths, and little food in the house. Mom went to work. So then we had shoes, somewhat better cloths, and still little food in the house.

There was no money for fun activities. We didn't skate, bowl or join in other activities. Whenever a group of kids was going skating I'd ask, "Can I go?" Soon I stopped asking. I felt so cheated. It really wasn't money it was all that and no hugs either. No soft warm whisper in your ear saying, "I'm glad you're home." The good feelings were so few and far between it didn't seem real. I felt like I was in a daze.

Once my grandfather took my sister and I to the circus. I was happy about going. I was looking forward to it. The day came. I was numb. We went to the circus. I felt nothing. I remember thinking, "Is that all there is. I thought it would be better." My grandfather bought me some cotton candy. When I got home I thanked my grandfather for taking me to the circus. But I mopped about so my mother kept asking me what was wrong. "Are you so ungrateful that he took you that you mope?" No. As it turned out I had a fever. My family then proceeded to be angry with my grandad. Blaming my illness on too much junk food. I don't believe one order of cotton candy made me sick. I believe I was sick from repressed emotions. The doctor came to our house and could find nothing wrong.

My grandmother would occasionally invite our family to dinner but never when my uncles or cousins were there. They were all college bred, ran in different circles, climbed the right social ladders. But my dad was a trucker, a race car driver, and my mother was a waitress and we did not fit. (This is the interpretation we heard from our parents. But as of this date August 1, 1994 I have come to believe it was for other reasons which were not exposed at that time.)

My parents were both hurt and felt rejected. They were wrapped up in their own problems. I watched. I saw their pain. I cried inside, "why aren't we good enough," my pain. I wanted to scream at them. I wanted to say, "It feels the same way over here." But no one noticed.

A little child coming from a poor family that has no money for curtains is asked, "What's a curtain?" does he know? No, he doesn't.

A child from a dysfunctional family is asked, "what is a loving family?' He doesn't know. "What does love behave like?" He doesn't know. He has seen anger and strife. True that most abusive parents do love their children, however, they either weren't capable of giving love or they didn't know how to show love. But what is modeled in the home doesn't look or feel like love. Since we can't get inside their head how do we know?

As an adult I know that even people that love each other argue. As a child I did not know. When my parents argued all I knew was fear.

My daughter witnessed several brutal events in my life at age three. I and my children made a new life. I remarried and feel that I have a good marriage. My daughter in now 21 years old. But recently when my husband and I argued my daughter shyly came in my room crying. "Oh, MaMa," she said. "You, and dad aren't getting a divorce, are you?" I held her and said, "dear, everyone argues sometimes." My dear daughter is now facing her abandonment needs. I'm happy she can do it now. Improve! Heal!

When we are from a dysfunctional family we have tunnel vision, black spots, we cannot see what others wee without trying. Because of what seems to be uncaring parents our thinking patterns are different. I married a rageaholic because I was use to rage. I thought, "So what else is new?" I didn't think I could do better. There were no choices for me, not in my mind. Now I have learned better. There are people in this world that love me for just who I am, some women, some men. In fact I have a lot of friends that are men. True friends, no threat to my husband at all.

Yes, love can be healthy. Love does not have to hurt. Love feels safe and good. With true love comes the ability to resolve conflicts, not ignore or pretend them away. We can have good friends and be a good friend. We can do work we enjoy.

We can ,"draw close to God," result, "he will draw close to you."

When we realize the above we are working out our deprivation needs. Our dysfunctional is very real. As a child adult we knew how to make the most out of it. I saved my money. I learned how to make a meal out of nothing. How has this affected me today? As long as there is food in my cabinets and refrigerator I don't even care if I eat or not, until recently anyway. I didn't care about food most of my life. I had learned it was not good to worry about it. Being hungry was painful. So I wasn't hungry. I gained weight because I didn't eat enough. Every time I'd start a diet I felt choked with all the food I had to eat to lose weight.

Then I started counseling. We never talked about these issues but after five or six weeks I wasn't feeling so guilty. I didn't realize what it was at the time but I started wanting to eat.

One evening I said, "You know what I'm hungry for...? My family all started to laugh. "What's wrong?" "Oh nothing mom, " they said. The next night I said, "hey let's get some pizza," again they start to laugh. My daughter who couldn't contain it anymore said, "Mom, it's just that we've never heard you say, 'I'm hungry/' what happened?" I realized I felt good.

In relationship to my father and candy. Many years after the incident described in the first of this chapter, this time I was 17 not 6, he came home on Halloween day with a grocery bag full of candy. We all dashed for the kitchen. His statement was, "this candy is not for you. It is for the trick or treaters." No we did not go out halloweening. We gave candy out to the halloweeners at our father's insistence. But for ourselves there was no candy. And when seventeen it felt just like when I was six. He cares more about them than us.

BECOMING THANKFUL

Is the glass half empty or half full? I always thought it was half empty. Since we're making changes let's change that too! The glass is half full. Here again our associations help. My husband who always looks for the positive started rubbing off on me. Pretty soon I was saying, Hey, I came out of the grocery store with a dollar left," instead of saying, "you know I spent$...... and I only have $.98 left what can I do with that?"

A friend of mine bought a new sweater. She paid about $70 for her sweater. We showed up at the same place with the same sweater. I bought mine at a rummage sale. I paid $2.00. I was so proud of myself. I hardly ever pay more than five dollars for anything and I have an abundance of cloths. Pretty good for a little girl with holes in her shoes and a couple of outfits to wear. What do I do with the money I save? I plan a budget. I have taken swimming lessons, my children swam before they walked, dancing lessons, college courses, German classes, redecorated my home, taken vacations. All the things I always wanted. I'm not saying rummage saling can do all that. I'm saying that life without fun caused us to be deprived. Many continued their state of deprivation for the rest of their lives. Fun is a natural course of events in our life. Have fun. If you have to do it on a shoestring, do it anyway. Pitch a tent. Pack a cooler. Make it fun to eat a picnic lunch in a beautiful area instead of complaining the only way you get to do anything is to sleep in a tent. You can't afford to eat in a restaurant. Enjoy the beauty of the outdoors and the company you are with.

Spending money on myself has gotten easier over the years. I allowed myself a small amount each week to spend on myself. This I did when in the process of a divorce. I had two preschoolers. Little financial help and no emotional support. Something inside of me said, "I count. Do this for yourself." I allowed myself $1.00 a week, many years ago. The first week was new makeup. The second, a necklace. I was feeling better. I was learning I needed to count with myself. I now have no trouble spending money, balance is what we are looking for. I'm still careful. I still buy sales. But this is the true me. I still know the best buy in town but I spend some on me and some on others. I feel good when I buy for others. I feel great when I buy for me.

Another really great thing I did for myself several weeks after starting therapy was to buy a different car. I always wanted a LaBaron. Now I have it. Something else that is great is that I bought it without help. Why Not!

I grew up in a family of mechanics. I know about cars. I showed up at the dealer by my lonesome, picked out the car, took it for a test drive. The sales man talked through most of the drive. Then said, "you're awful quite." "Shhh!" I said. "I'm listening to hear when the car shifts gears." Boy, did I see one surprised salesman. I looked under where the car had set for oil, and checked the oil, checked out the body for puttied in spots, checked the tires to see if they needed rotating, then since the place was ready to close I told the man I really needed to see how the car performed on the highway. He agreed to let me take it for the night. One last thing I asked him if he would start the car while I watched the exhaust, so I could tell if it was burning oil or not.

Well, I bought the car, but I did make him earn his commission. It was a LaBaron and that's what I wanted. A far cry from driving an old ugly green car I didn't like. Yes, we can change. I am changing. It feels good.

I believe the moral of this story is: If we believe we deserve good things, we can act in a way that we can have some good things. If we believe we deserve having good people that love us with no strings we will have it. We will have it because we won't settle for anyone who comes along because we don't think we can do better.

Our deprivation years have served us well. The skills we acquired to get through those years help us even now to have things a little better, even materially. But we need not continue them. This is within my ability to change. Just because we lived through deprivation years doesn't mean we have to keep playing the role. My deprivation of the past can, however, help me to be thankful for what I have today. We need not continue role playing, rebel roles, good girl roles, the star, and the clown roles. We have changed them for our being. I need not exchange them if those things are part of the true me. I do however have a different motive. I've given up being a clown because of the need to hide. But I still clown. I love clownaroundery. My being has given up:

Being a caretaker to become a caring person.

Being a good girl to doing what I believe to be right because I want to not because I need to.

The star has become an average person. How good it is. The pressure is off. I can be average.

The clown still clowns but I don't need to to get the attention I need. I don't clown around to hide from the sorrow I feel. I clown around because I feel good.

Being grateful has lifted our hearts. We can improve other areas of our life a little at a time. It is a process. We were angry. We were deprived. We were angry because we were deprived. We are learning to process our anger. Learn how our deprivation can help us now to be grateful for what we have and not continue the course of deprivation. In large we reduce our anger by setting appropriate boundaries. Appropriate boundaries reduce our anger and deprivation. Another paradoxical recovery. So be it. I need not deprive myself when I know I am a worthy person. I am not their victim. I will not be their victim. I protect myself from being their victim by knowing how to set and enforce boundaries.

BOUNDARIES

Boundaries are our lines, our limits, this is our personal territory or space. I will not allow any one to manipulate my mind or emotions, my right to think and feel as I think and feel. I am open to suggestions. I can use feedback, information, to grow. This is different. Feedback is for the purpose of deciphering our thoughts and feelings. Not allowing others to tell us what to think and what to feel. Those who manipulate are doing so in order to control us so they will will safe, competent, and/or powerful . This fills a need in them. They would keep us needing them as long as we let them. Our boundaries are like an emotional fence. Fences are for the purpose of protection. No one can see our invisible fence but it is there. It is there to protect us. To honor our right to be a unique individual not to be a copy of someone else. Without our fence we are open to trespassers. Those who have not the right to be in our territory. When we are born our mind is like a blank slate. What we are exposed to is what we learn. Our healthy parents teach us healthy respect, boundaries. We establish boundaries. Our self respect yields more self respect. An emotionally healthy wife would not take on the blame for an abusive husband. I f we had unhealthy parents we were supposed to be like them. We had no idea where they end and we begin, no boundaries, or weak boundaries, maybe boundaries with holes in them. Our abusive background, our lack of emotional strokes, our possible neglect in infancy, the lack of nurturing, lack of appropriate limits and discipline produced a person who is open to violation. If our boundaries have holes in them we need to repair it. Now!

Some built brick walls to defend themselves. Walls of denial. Denial thus becomes our protection. Denial refuses to let us know we need to set boundaries. Nothing is wrong here. Reality says, everything is wrong here.

Lack of boundaries are;

1. Family members coming into the bathroom while you are in the bathroom.

2. Family members that walk around the house in their underclothing. Whether or not it is sexual. It is dysfunctional.

3. Having no private area to change cloths.

4. Family members sharing your private problems without your permission.

5. Not having the right to say what I feel I need to say for my own protection.

6. Being told to ignore kids in school that bully you. Parents do not know how to be they children's advocate. They do not know any other advice in how to deal with conflict other than avoid i t or fight them. So ignore them is usually the advice we get.

7. When we are expected to fill the role as an adult as a child. We could not say, "This is too much for me.'

8. Being neglected as a child. The message was, "you don't matter enough for me to take time with you."

9. Being beaten with canes, electric cords, hangers, brooms, chairs, pots, pans or whatever was in their hand when they lost control.

10. Punishment was inappropriate to our mistake.

11. If we took care of those who were supposed to take care of us, parents.

I had been role playing all my life. I was the caretaker. How could I establish boundaries. I was taking care of others people feelings not my own. I cannot caretake their feelings and set boundaries. The two are diametrically opposed.

Our bond with our original caregiver determines how we will bond and go about bonding with others. Our boundaries will determine how we allow ourselves to fix. Who we allow into our territory and who we do not know how to stop from coming into our territory when we don't want them there. Boundaries are our means of protection. Without boundaries we will be afraid of relationships. Too many boundaries produce no relationships in our life. We pull away out of fear of being hurt. When we have healthy boundaries other people are comfortable around us. Those who attempt to control will not be comfortable around us. This is okay. This is yet another protection from their controlling. We will not be comfortable around those who would control, invade our territory. Controlling people feel it is their right to tell us what to think and feel. Afterall their care. But what does healthy caring have to do with telling another person what to think? What we are endeavoring to do is to learn to establish good boundaries. Learn how to flex with a situation and not forsake ourself. I do not want anyone to step on my boundary nor will I deliberately step on theirs. If I step on their boundary I would appreciate being told. I may do so without knowing this is your boundary so please tell me. This is healthy, balanced, functional boundaries. Knowing my right to have rights and still acknowledging your rights to think and feel differently than I. Your right to have different boundaries than I.

The Idea of setting boundaries became very fearful to me. Little did I know I was already setting and enforcing new boundaries. I only knew I was angry. I said, "I don't think so." "This one I will handle myself." "Please stay out of it." "I've considered information available on this subject and I have decided to..." "I heard what you said. I disagree." "I think it best if we drop this conversation." "I would appreciate it if we could agree to disagree." All communicate our new boundary to the other person in a few words. Do not spell out a lot of details. We want to leave no doubt as to what we are asking from them. Nor do we want them to be unclear about what we will or will not allow in this relationship from this point on. If they disagree they are free to say so. Each of us then have the right to detach from the other if that is what it takes to stand by our boundaries. We will be tested when we set boundaries. Those who are used to controlling us will be angry. They do not realize why we are changing . They are aware of the changes. They have not settled their own dysfunctional issues. They perceive our changes as a personal affront to them. In setting our boundaries we must be prepared to stand by them regardless of the reaction of other people. "When I accept my limits and enforce my boundaries I am free to be me. I believe in order to set effective boundaries I must acknowledge my limits. I need to acknowledge the part of me that says, "I can't stand it." "I hate it when." "I'm angry about." One of the things I was angriest about was how often I felt anger after I started recovery. After I had finished my business I found myself to be angry often. This was very upsetting to me. I always thought, "I don't get angry easily." Now I found I did. Recovery is not about not getting angry. Recovery is about knowing what we feel. If I get upset about little things than I know the solution. The solution always rest in two things,

1. setting appropriate boundaries
2. detaching from what I cannot control.

Boundaries and detachment go hand in hand. Another paradox of recovery. When I set and enforce a boundary I learn where I need to detach. When I detach I have greater strength to enforce my boundaries. My boundaries in effect say, this is what I will or will not allow others to do to me. I can give an ultimatum. I personally do not feel this is the best solution. I feel it is best saved as a last resort. If I must I can. I can say to another, "you cannot drink and live in this house." I know at this point the other person has a choice. My ultimatum will not cause them to stop drinking unless they see the benefit to their own life. They may choose to stop drinking. They may not. If they don't I must be prepared to live with what I stated. "They cannot live in this house." My boundary is for me to improve the quality of my life. I know life's quality improves if one does not live with an alcoholic or other compulsive person. Ultimatums are great risk. To give an ultimatum in the hopes of getting the other person to stop drinking or whatever is not recovery. It is control. If I give an ultimatum and cannot enforce what I said I have made my situation worse. I needed to get angry to start setting boundaries. Soon I found that I needn't stay angry. Boundary setting had become fun. It was and is a thrill to say, "No sir, not here in my house." "Excuse me, I think not."

Boundary setting is about learning how to take care of our needs. This we do as an integral part of being the true us. No matter where I am or who I am with. We know we deserve to have the right to make decisions about our life without being in fear of what others think. I learned to say, "I will not be in any friendship or relationship where I am the only one working on this relationship. Your boundaries are important to me. Mine must be important to you. If this is not the case it is not a relationship."

I was confused and nervous about boundary setting but as I attended my first Alanon meeting the issue became clear. The speaker that night spoke of boundaries and limits. I came home and wrote the chapter GOALS, BOUNDARIES, AND LIMITS for my first book PROFILE OF ABUSE. My eyes had been opened wide. I learned to say, "I would like to be your friend but I will not be friends with anyone who curses me, calls me names, or lies to me. I will not be verbally or any other way abused." it felt good! I learned to say, "I cannot be friends under these circumstances. I've learned how to say no without guilt. Say no even if you feel guilty. You already feel guilty so you have nothing to lose.

I needed to set boundaries. In time my new boundaries gained me respect, respect from those I had detached from, new friendships, better friendships. However, what I gained immediately was self respect. This was not so hard. This was enlightening. The more we put into practice setting and enforcing our boundary the easier it will become. However we may find some difficulty setting boundaries when our circumstances change. We may find ourselves in turmoil about where and when to set a boundary under this situation. If we feel bad, if it bothers us this is where we need a boundary. Forsaking a boundary may come about because we failed to communicate our boundary to others. I remember a woman who said she set boundaries in her head. She didn't realize she must communicate them to others.

Recovery is about communication. We need to communicate our boundaries to others. We need to communicate we have every intent of standing by what we said. We need to communicate our anger. We need to communicate that we are doing our best to handle our anger appropriately and that we find this is best done by communicating to them why we are angry and what does not work in this relationship as well as what we want from this relationship. These are my needs, wants, and desires. I am telling you in the hopes we can work out solutions to keep this relationship in tact. When I do so I know you have needs, wants, and desires. I am also interested in yours. Let's work together to honor each other and each other's right to their needs, wants, and desires. This I call a relationship.

The above paragraph is healthy boundary setting. It is not selfishness. While we are learning to take care of ourselves we are also learning to show respect in every relationship. Respect simply means I try to understand how you feel even if I don't agree I don't try to make you me.

When we stand by healthy boundary setting we will not relapse into a setback. We will grow. Our confidence level will grow. We are now becoming functional. The fears we had about boundaries will disappear. As abused children we became hypervigalant, always watchful, observing, analyzing every situation for potential danger. Now we can use this skill of observation to let us know we can trust what we can see, hear and how we feel about it. Based on information and our feelings about that information we can make good decisions about boundaries. We will know if it is safe or not and what to do to protect myself. My protection is wrapped up in my boundaries.

Boundaries and limits are directly related to each other. When I set limits I know where to set a boundary. When I set and enforce my boundary I am more aware of my limits. It feels good to be responsible for myself and still care about other people. I have learned not to overcommitt. A direct result of establishing boundaries.

I have only been able to effectively set boundaries since I began my family of origin work, also called finishing my business. I experienced growing self esteem. I learned how to deal with my feelings. I broke all the family rules that had kept me controlled. I talked about it. I detached where necessary. I found the causes for my shame. If I feel shame I cannot set boundaries. I found the causes of my shame only to find it never was my shame. Whenever I felt good I felt guilt. Guilt for the dreaded sin of arrogance. Now I have come to understand I have never been arrogant. I can feel a healthy sense of accomplishment and not think I am better than another.

I can feel my own feelings because every feeling I have is not tied into my shame. If I feel good about myself I need not be shamed. If I do something wrong, I'm okay. I'm normal. I goof up. What I did may not be okay. I can set my boundary because I am able to talk about how I feel and why I feel it. I am not ashamed of what happened to me. I am not those events. Our shame kept us in their control. As our self esteem grows, as we build healthy relationships, boundaries become easier, Easier to see, easier to set, easier to enforce. Boundaries is one of the most important skills to master if we are going to heal.

BOUNDARY SETTING CONVERSATIONS

Your sister; "Let's go visit mom."

Yourself; " Whenever we visit mom I get behind in everything I have to do.

Your Sister; "You don't like going with me?"

Yourself: "NO, what I meant to say is that although I like going I do not keep up with what I have to do. This week I am way behind schedule. I will have to pass.

Friend; Can you help me move Saturday?
Yourself: I can't this Saturday. I've already promised my wife to spend the day with her.
Friend: Surely Susie will understand.
Yourself: I think I need to keep my word to Susie. Say if you still need help on Sunday I can help you for a few hours.
Friend: I really need your help Saturday.
Yourself; Saturday is taken. But what if I call you Sunday morning and see if you still need help?

In general boundary setting statements are those that are direct statements which clearly let another person know what we can and what we cannot do. We can show empathy for their situation and still stand by our boundaries. Ex.

Friend; Gee Dee, I'm in an awful jam. I need a thousand dollars to..... Could you lend it to me for just a few weeks?

Dee; I can see what a jam you're in but I don't feel comfortable lending out that much money.

If I wish I can add and explanation but my rule of thumb is; if I feel guilty, if I feel I must give an explanation to not feel guilty in this situation then I don't give an explanation. It was this method that helped me learn how to say no without feeling guilty. I will add an explanation if I feel the need. If I feel no one is trying to guilt trip me and if I feel my explanation will not be invalidated by the other person. In effect I consider who I am talking with and how I know they perceive my rights. To my one friend I always say, "Fay, I can't today because....." She always says, "I see why you feel that way." No problem. To another person I never give an explanation. This person is the one that says, "Surely you can do that another time I really need your help." I refuse to supply another person ammunition.

When dealing with very difficult people we will need to use a method called the broken record. We in effect say the same thing over and over until even the most stubborn will get the point.

Salesperson; We have the greatest deal ever on our subscriptions.
Yourself; Thank you but I'm not interested.
Salesperson; Our sale gives you a savings of 30% off the...
Yourself; That does sound like a good deal but I am not interested.
Salesperson; Are you a reader?
Yourself: Yes, I am but I am not interested.
Salesperson: One subscription could get you back into the reading mode which one would you like to subscribe to today?
Yourself: I do read. Today I am not interested.
Salesperson; How about trying....
Yourself; I appreciate you have a hard job but I am not interested in a subscription. I wish you all success. Thank you. Goodbye.

It is important to give the real reason or no reason for the boundary you have expressed. You are not required to tell another why. For example;

A friend wants to borrow your car. You say, "Gee my insurance won't cover you." Your friend says, "My insurance covers me no matter what I drive." Now you are stuck.

Wouldn't it be more accurate, more truthful, and more effective to say, "I can see the spot you're in but I don't lend out my car." This gives less fuel for them to invalidate your reason, your boundary, about not lending out your car. They may say in return, "I have insurance that covers me if that's what you're worried about." Your reply, "No, I just have a policy that says, I don't lend out my car. If you can go after I get off of work I will take you."

By adding on the last statement you have showed your reasonableness. You have showed your caring. Only make this offer if you feel you can do so and feel good about helping your friend. If the offer is out of guilt you will still be stuck in the same dysfunction.

OVERALL BOUNDARY SETTING STATEMENTS

I'd like to help but my schedule is too full this week. Would next week work for you?

In that case I will have to pass?

I can't help this time but I would like to next time, will you let me know a few days ahead of time.

I see the spot you're in however I too am.....

i see the spot you're in. This time however I chose to pass.

I can't help you with this problem but I know someone that you could ask, see what he thinks about.......

Thank you for thinking of me but I am not able to work that into my schedule at this time.

No, I cannot take care of your dog while you are away at school. Please look for someone else ahead of time.

I already have plans for that day.

Thank you, but I am too tired.

No, I do not feel like making love. I would like to spend some time together. Why don't we go to a movie.

Honey, could we just hold each other tonight.

I'm sorry I will not be able to work overtime.

Yes, I understand how important this is to you. Let me know if I can help in any other way.

I understand this is important to you I wish you well.

No, I cannot buy you a lottery ticket. It is against my personal beliefs.

I need to tell you that I was upset about.....

Excuse me, I think not.

No Way!

I must go. No I cannot stay longer. Then do what you say.

As we see some statements are stronger than others. If someone suggestingly puts there hand on my shoulder, I think removing their hand and saying, "NO WAY!" is appropriate. Our boundaries are protected while they are still enforceable. This is always easiest done in the bud. Yes, nip it in the bud.

VERBAL JUDO

Healing is hard work. We must learn new skills. Skills we will use for the rest of our life. We will heal and stay healed only when we learn the art of using these tools.

One of the most effective tools at our disposal is establishing our boundaries. Dr David Burns in his book Feeling good talks about a skill called verbal judo. Verbal judo is the light of my life. Verbal judo is the ability to talk back to someone who is angry with us, insulting us, and do it in a way that does not inflame the situation nor does it put us in the position where we allow them to verbally or otherwise abuse us.

A similar definition is verbal judo is the ability to speak up for myself even when under fire from a difficult person, without throwing insults or accusations. Verbal Judo is a few skills that will help us to deal with difficult people. None of these steps are difficult. At first we will have to make a conscious effort to think about them and how to put them into practice. With time it gets easier. Each time we are able to do it our self esteem builds. After 6 months or so we can look back and see we are indeed a different person. This is an art. There are several different approaches.

First we develop empathy. Recovery is about empathy. But learning about our thoughts and feelings we have learned empathy for ourselves. By learning how to listen to ourself we too have learned how to listen to others. Put the same ideas to work. Listen. Not with an ear of judgment. Listen to what is said while trying not to be judgmental. Listen to the feelings in their words. We need not feel sympathy for them. It does mean that our thoughts are cognitive. We are attempting to see the whole picture, not just our side. Not just theirs. Even if they are criticizing us they may be right. They may be wrong, or somewhere in the middle. I always thought I was doing this by shutting my mouth and listening to them. Now upon learning about verbal judo I was infuriated. Listen. Listening does not mean you are agreeing or believing what they say. Listen with the view of understanding where they are coming from. It's called putting ourselves in their shoes. I thought for many years this is what I was doing. But I was in reality doing was listening to their problem and them putting my personality into their shoes and sizing up what they should do. Really putting ourselves into their shoes is to hear what they have to say. Understanding their personality will react different in this situation than I do. Trying not to judge their reaction because it is different than mine. Really try to understand why they react the way they do. Now comes the important aspect of verbal judo. They have wound down. I do not try to defend myself by attacking the things they said. Notice this; I did not say I do not try to defend myself. I said. I do not try to defend myself by attacking the things they said. This is different than dysfunction. This is not standing there taking verbal abuse until I can take no more and then making up some excuse to leave. This is only a different way to defend myself. I am practicing standing by my boundaries and by use of verbal judo I will be able to handle difficult people and situations that arise.

Verbal Judo is about defending myself. We use new skills to do so. We have set boundaries. We are endeavoring to stand by them. They will push a little harder. We are now able to defend ourselves instead of giving in to them and their control. They will get the idea.

We have allowed them to have their say. Now we do not pick apart what they have said about us. We can say, "I'm sorry that you feel that way." "I'm sorry there was a problem between us." This in no way implies guilt on our part. At this point we have opened the way for a conversation not a battle. We can now ask them a series of questions. These questions are designed to get the specifics of what it is that they feel I do wrong.

SAMPLE CONVERSATION

You: You are so stupid.

Me; What is it that I do that makes you feel that I am stupid.

You; It's everything you say and do. You talk too much. You wear your makeup stupid. You are overweight. Your insensitive and selfish.

Me: Maybe we need to talk. I would like you to be specific. What is it I have done or said that has upset you? What did I say that sounded insensitive to you? What gave you the impression I am more concerned about myself than others?

You: When I tried to talk with you you did most of the talking and I did not feel that you cared about me at all. And sometimes it feels that you are always in such a hurry that I don't think you listen at all.

Me: So I came across to you that I want to do all the talking and did not want to listen to you, even being in too much of a hurry to listen.

You: Yes, and that's not the only time. You have done this quite often.
Me: Okay. I see why you would be upset. I think anybody would. If they felt someone else always does the talking and doesn't listen to them.

What are the skills involved in the above dialogue?

1. empathic listening
2. paraphrasing back what I think I heard
3. asking for specific's
4. Agreeing where I can
5. Letting pass what I feel inappropriate.

What is accomplished by doing so?

1. kept things cool
2. I gain insight into the other person.

Did the fact that things stayed cool and I listened and asked questions mean that I was admitting to doing such and such? No!

If we think the criticism is unfounded ask specific questions? This allows you to know where the other person is coming from and with what you will be dealing. Ask,

1. How did you offend them?
2. What was it I did?
3. How often have I done this?
4. What else about me don't you like?

This takes a big person. It will be worth the effort. Somewhere in the process we may find a grain of truth. Now we have learned about ourselves. We can grow. Learn from it. Change it if we see the need.

Second in the use of verbal judo is what is referred to as disarming the critic. When we are being assaulted verbally we can do several things. We can hurl back- chances are you won't feel too good about yourself later. This is venting. This is also verbal abuse on our part to another.

We can run away. This is not recovery. We have learned not to run. Not to live in denial. This is about learning how to continue our recovery in a way that allows us to maintain and build our self esteem as well as enforce our boundaries. Doing so in a way that will benefit even those who are not aware we are working a recovery program. W e will also be role modeling what recovery is and how it has improved the quality of our life to those who think at this time that they do not need recovery. At some point in time they may join us.

The third thing we can do when we are being verbally accosted is to stay where you are and disarm them. How do we go about this? I find something in what they said to agree with. Ex. I can say, "Yes the last time we talked I was in a hurry. It's possible I came across as not interested. That has been called to my attention by others. I assure you I did not intend to put you off."

This is not codependency. It is not dysfunction. As we become more and more functional and strive to live functionally we will find how much dysfunction we notice. Other people are not going to change their communication style to suit us. We are being functional by knowing how to handle these situations as they arise. We are giving to them what we ourselves needed to accomplish our growth. We are giving them our ear. Whether or not we agree we validate this is how you feel. I understand how you feel does not mean we agree. We simply see their side. We disarm or defuse the situation by verbalizing to them that we see why they feel as they do. Avoid sarcasm. We must speak the truth. If we do not understand simply state, "I am trying to understand why you are upset. It is possible I rushed away." On one occasion someone said to me, "Who's fault is that?" I said, "Mine." I could see their shoulders drop and tension being released. The other person was so shocked at my answer that they gave way to more reasonableness. A door for conversation opened that had not previously existed. If we made a mistake acknowledge it. This does not in any way admit that everything they say is true. Many years ago before I knew about functional and dysfunctional families or anything on this subject my ex-mother-in-law and I had a viscous quarrel. My then husband would always say to me, "What did you do to make a fight with my mother?" He never said, "What happened?" So he was insistence that I apologize to his mother while I felt she was the one who had overstepped her rights and I had taken it long enough. He and I fought for days. "You must apologize and that is all there is to it," he said. "I am taking you over to my mother's and you will apologize." We got in the car. I did not know what to do. I prayed for help while we were on our way there. When we got there I went into the house, her and I were alone, and I said, "I owe you an apology for screaming at you. I was wrong." Her reply, "but that's it. You have not changed your mind. You are going to keep doing things like you do. You haven't changed your mind at all, have you?" I was afraid but I was also angry. I stood tall and said, "No, I haven't." This brought on a whole new set of insults. I only said, "I came here to apologize for what I did wrong. I think it is wrong to scream at people and for that I have apologized. I do not feel we need to argue again because I came to apologize." My husband came in the room asking if I apologized. His mother explained that I had but only for screaming at her and nothing else. What was my everything else? It was having different ideas than they. It was speaking up when I was tired of being insulted. Now the fight began again. Him demanding I apologize to his mother. I walked out. Walked home. Changed the locks and told him to live with his mother.

Yes I was very dysfunctional. But somewhere in the above I received an answer that was functional. I got it only from prayer. I apologized for my part. "I'm sorry I screamed at you." We need not take the blame for their dysfunction or their perceptions.

I believe in most cases people will accept our apology. We acknowledge what we did. After that if they continue to berate we can use what is referred to as the broken record method. We simply say the same thing again. As they continue I can say, "I'm sorry, we had a problem. If I was wrong I apologize."

Following is an example of finding a point to agree with. I use this example regularly in a class I teach.

Teacher; You are not the best student in my class. I do not know why you bothered to take the class. You take over the class whenever possible. You took this class to get attention.

Student; What gives you the impression I took this class to get attention?

Teacher; You don't participate. You try to run the show. You don't do the homework assignments.

Student: It's true that I may have spoken up without being called on. It is also true that I did not do the homework. Do you feel I should not speak out so much?

Teacher; Do what you want! You will anyway. You love messing up my class.

Student; I am aware I need to work on that. Do you have any suggestions. This is difficult for me.

Teacher; I give up. You win.

Lets's identify some techniques this student used. The teacher was totally out of control. The student listened, asked for specifics, did not retaliate with what he does not do. That is not true. The student acknowledged what the teacher said that was true and left the rest pass. The student then asked for helpful ideas for him to improve.

I believe it is a good idea to practice with a friend. If you can't do this or feel uncomfortable about it then you can write imaginary dialogues between you and someone that is angerly speaking to you or down at you.

Important point: do not try to prove untrue the things you disagree with. It is a natural reaction to defend yourself. This is a mistake. Think of verbal Judo as a different way to defend yourself. When we attack back in our defense the whole situation become explosive. It is quite the opposite when someone responses with empathy and disarms what you said then you feel listened to. You feel respected. So do they. This will not come automatically. It's like everything else it will take conscious effort. We will want to jump in with old behaviors. We can learn from it. Afterward analyze what you think your mistakes are and then maybe you can practice writing dialogues. The advantage of practicing ahead of time is that you are not thrown off base when the real event happens. Don't expect it to come out just like your written dialogue. We do not write it out to plan the outcome. We not not write it out to find a way to get them to..... in the conversation. We do not practice ahead of time to control the person or the situation. One trademark of dysfunction is that many plan their words to strike the heart. They plan how to manipulate or control the other person's responses. This is different. Control is not our goal. We practice ahead of time so we are prepared to handle our end of the situation in a way that we prefer. Usually what most people do in any type of conflict is to react. Afterward they say I wish I would have, I should have, If only I could take it back or do it over. This is our chance. The things we wish we would have done are our true self speaking. When we are overwhelmed our controlling child takes over. Recovery is about releasing the power of the controlling child.

The things I wish I would have done, the way I would have preferred to act, our true self can only gain the power, confidence, and ability to act in times of conflict if we practice, think about, make a conscious decision to carry it out. When we mess up look at our mistakes, instead of saying I should have...... which I believe to be a guilt trip that only perpetuates negative thinking and negative actions. I have all but eliminated should from my vocabulary. I say the next time I will.... I have now turned a shame producing statement into a confidence boosting statement. I make a conscious decision to carry out different and more effective behaviors. I have given up control. My preparation is only to better equip myself to act in a legitimate way. To act the way I prefer to act rather than letting other people and situations control my reactions.

We have listened with empathy. We have asked specific questions? We have disarmed the situation where possible.. The next step in verbal judo is feedback and negotiation.

Let's assume your critic is totally wrong. How can we verbalize this to them in a nondestructive way?

1. express our point of view as objectively as possible and also express it's possible we might be wrong. Use I statements. Say I think, I feel, rather than you did. I can say,

Here's how I feel about this situation.

What I think is.....

How I see this situation is....

I can certainly see why you are upset. I think the problem here is....

2. Make the conflict into a conflict of facts or even opinions. We are in effect agreeing to disagree. We are not defaming another because they are different than us. The prime premise of dysfunction.

3. Do not make it into a conflict of personalities. I am not better than you because I choose to handle this situation this way instead of the way you are doing it.

4. Do not name call.

Sometimes the conflict is a matter of taste. Such as in clothing or makeup. One person says, 'too much eye shadow." Another might say, "don't wear eyeliner." Yet another might say, "Oh, you didn't wear your eye liner today. You look so much better with it."

If this proves to be a constant problem I can assertively address the issue. I can state, "I can see your point, however I have found that this is the way I best like my makeup."

It doesn't hurt to compromise. If it is a genuine compromise not a giving in to please. But do this only after you have applied the empathy and disarming technique. Do not compromise your position in the heat of their dysfunction. Do not give control of your life to another. Even if another person gives me an ultimatum I can choose to follow the ultimatum if I think it is the best thing for my life at this time. I will not however give to them my power. In this case, if I decide to do as they wished in their ultimatum statement I will make it clear to them I have chosen to do this because I think it is best for me at this time. I do not turn my power over to them.

What if it turns out you were the one that was in the wrong? The person who criticizes you is right. You will earn the respect of the other person and even yourself by admitting it. In this case;

1. agree with the criticism.

2. thank the person for telling you. We need not address the method they used to tell us. It is not important whether or not we like them, or the manner in which they addressed our fault. What is important is that we have learned something about ourselves that we need to know and work on for personal improvement.

3. apologize for any pain you may have caused.

This is hard. It takes a very mature person. Think about how you will feel about yourself when you have accomplished it. You will be able to pat yourself on the back with a well deserved, "JOB WELL DONE."

In addition you will have gained a considerable amount of respect from the other person. Haven't we all heard someone say, "I was shocked. He listened. He admitted he was wrong. Maybe I was wrong about him. He's okay." We have just greatly increased the chances that in the future our differences with that person will be handled in a much more respectful manner.

We have just learned how to defend ourselves without bringing ourself down to the level of venting and hurting others. We have learned to empathize, disarm and then negotiate. We can admit when we are wrong. We can act as though we have tons of self respect even if we don't. This is not the false front put on by dysfunction. This is priming the pump.

If we act in a self respecting way we learn to respect ourself for what we have just accomplished. This gives us more confidence for the next trial some situation. Yes, I can do this. And we do. Our respect for others is demonstrated while we grow in respect for ourselves.

Verbal Judo is a very important skill that helps us to handle even the more difficult situations with self respect and confidence. It is a skill used in becoming an assertive person. We are able to be assertive because,

1. we have sorted through our causes of shame.
2. we are learning verbal expressions that are effective communication skills.

Neither verbal judo or assertiveness training is a tool for manipulation and control. The aggressive person sees every challenge as a potential attack on his person. While the assertive person knows what they think or feel. The assertive person does not need to apologize for expressing their feelings and thoughts. They are not manipulated by false guilt. The assertive person does not expect others to forsake their rights so they can get theirs. Verbal judo then is not a tool to control the outcome. Verbal judo is simply a dignified way to response to the verbal overreacting of others. We keep our dignity and allow them to return to theirs. Verbal judo is the most effective tool we have in the use of fighting fair rules which we will discuss next.

ACCURATE COMMUNICATION

What would each of us consider the most important factor in any relationship? How many conflicts we have is not as important as how a conflict is handled when there is conflict. Whether it is many or few. Most of us have either been striving not to have conflict or live on the adrenaline high produced by conflict.

Fighting fair is a major accomplishment in our life. In fact learning to fight fair is a recent development to the whole human race. Our generation is learning new skills that if applied will benefit ourselves as well as the security or our children. Not long before I started therapy my husband and I had a major difference of opinion with a local merchant. We left a message for him to call us. This he did. We explained why we did not feel we owed such and such. The way this man handled himself was very functional and according to all verbal judo and fight fair rules. At the time neither of us were aware of this information. I later commented to my husband that the conversation was unusual and how nice he was even though he was angry. Neither of us had ever seen anger handled appropriately before this incident. This must be why I remember it. This we can do for others. We might make a difference.

In the past it was thought that we do our best not to fight. But when people fell into an argument everyone felt like a failure and few people knew how to resolve the issues at hand. Those who are attempting to be mature argue or try to refrain from arguing then apologize and start over. Issues however never get settled. The same issue or problem is fought about for many years. Children grow up in an atmosphere where nothing ever gets settled therefore they do not expect to settle differences in their relationships. Thus they learn that life's problems cannot be settled why bring this up? The cycle of dysfunction continues for yet another generation.

What we are learning is that problems can be settled. It is worth while to bring them up. We can say, "this is what I need." We can address the problem of the present without rehashing old wounds. We learn also that we can be forgiven when we make mistakes. We learn everyone makes mistakes. In the dysfunctional family we feel nothing we ever do is good enough. We feel we must cover our mistakes or we may admit to our mistakes and spend most of our life trying to please others to make up for our mistakes. Learning about fighting fair helps us to see issues are settled. We are forgiven for our mistakes. This we learn through seeing things are settled not hung onto and fought about for many years.

Fighting fair allows both parties to express their feelings in a respectful manner while not dodging the issues they need to settle. Before doing so it is important to learn a few things about men and woman's communication styles. Whatever gender we are we are better able to work at active listening when we understand the thinking process of the other party.

We will discuss active listening a little later in the chapter.

Relationships are about feelings. Men and women think through a different process. Debra Tannen authoress of YOU JUST DON'T UNDERSTAND WOMEN AND MEN IN CONVERSATION wrote that at about age 2-2 1/2 the developmental styles of girls and boys begin to show a difference.

Females talk their way through a thought process. A woman is talking to come to a solution. Also why women are more willing to ask for directions. Be they how to get somewhere or directions on how to communicate, how to.... Women use conversation as a way to negotiate closeness and intimacy. Talk is the essence of intimacy.

Males think out a problem then express the solution in usually a few sentences. Men see conversation as a competition. Men's conversation is goal oriented. If one man says, "I caught an 8" catfish the other day." The other man must tell about the time he caught the oldest grandad of them all. It must have been 36"s. Or he caught the biggest fish in the gulf. One man brags about his new girl and the other starts telling how ugly this guys last girlfriend was.

Women catch a small fish and the other woman will join in to tell about when she fishes all day and all she got was a little fish. Bonding and validation have taken place. Men compete with each other, women empathize and bond.

The woman is talking to draw close and men use it to compete or problem solve. So while she thinks talking will bring her closer to her husband the husband is wondering what her problem is.

Men express intimacy by doing things together.

Women express intimacy by talking. I remember a trip my husband and I took to Maine. I had decided not to play the radio or talk. Let him talk. See if he talks. He didn't. Three days on the road only brought on occasional, "I love you," with a pat on my leg. Sometimes a, "do you need a rest stop?" or "isn't it beautiful?" By the third day in the middle of the afternoon I was going nuts. I had not played the radio as that would have kept him from talking as he doesn't want to interrupt my music. I tell him I only play the music to keep from being bored. I'll turn it off anytime. So this trip no radio, no kids. I'm about to go crazy from the silence. My husband smiles lovingly at me pats my leg and said, "I love you," and I began to cry. "I've had enough. You say you don't talk at home because the kids always cut you off or you are tired. It's been three days and all you got to say is I love you. I haven't played the radio or talked. You have no competition. So why?"

His reply, "Gee I'm having a ball just being with you."

Me; "I'm not. What good is being with me if we don't share?"

That began of process of at least understanding. As I learned more about styles of communication between the genders I understood my husband more. We may not choose to communicate in their style however when we understand we will be less frustrated, more validated.

I also believe that I can adapt my style of communication considering the gender of the person I am speaking with. Men like direct statements. "I think I would like to go out of town for the weekend. I think I'm overworked and it would be a nice rest." Straight to the point. We will greatly increase the probability of being listened to.

When I am talking to a woman I can tell the little details of the story if it seems appropriate and time permits. Tell only the details that are pertinent to the point we are trying to make.

Conflicts between men and women come when the woman is talking about feelings and the man wants to rush to the solution. He does not talk through the problem. He has done or will do this in his head. All the while the woman is thinking, he isn't doing anything. He isn't saying anything. I'm sick of it.

This can be used to the best of both worlds if both parties will learn a few new skills. Communication is a few good skills and the willingness to learn them. The good news is: NONE OF THESE SKILLS ARE DIFFICULT TO LEARN.

Accurate Communication Skills

1. learn to express our feelings in "I statements". I think this is what is going on, I feel good about our trip. I think you need to work on your tone of voice.
2. understand differences in gender communication skills
3. learn active listening skills
4. learn and use fight fair rules when disagreements arise
5. use verbal judo to deal with difficult people
6. understand ourself and our feelings. If we do not understand ourself how can they.

All of these will be discussed within this chapter. Keep these things in mind. If you are female remember; he is not deliberately trying to cut me off. He is only acting male.

If you are male remember; she is not deliberately being long winded. She is being female. She is more emotional. Therefore there are more emotions to sort. Remember this; the more information I put into my computer the more time it takes for the computer to sort and organize that information. Females generally look at the broader scope of things. More information, more time to sort.

Each relationship must have certain qualities to make a commitment to making this relationship work. To make the relationship work we know we will conflict at times. Our goal is to handle these conflicts in a way that leaves everyone with their self respect and resolves not denies the issues. These qualities are;

1. moderate compatibility
2. clear communication- honest, open , and constructive.
3. How to resolve conflicts constructively.

If we do not as yet have these skills we only need want to learn and apply them in our lives.

To have good communication we have to be aware of our own feelings. We need to be able to take responsibility for our feelings positive and/or negative. We need to possess the ability to separate baggage. We as an assertive person do not try to manipulate or control others by false blaming, criticism, and guilt. We all became aware in our school days of the scientific law that says, "to every action there is an equal and opposite reaction." Blaming begets blaming. Blaming is a form of controlling. We in breaking the cycle of dysfunction are releasing control.

Our process of recovery is wrapped up in the two most important words in the English language, they are ACCURATE COMMUNICATION. Accurate communication prevents much pain. And most of what is not prevented is healed when we accurately communicate.

To communicate I must first listen.

REASONS TO LISTEN

1. communication is improved through listening
2. listening helps us to learn self restraint
3. Listening lessens arguments.
4. We demonstrate we care when we listen.
5. We feel more connected to the world and things around us when we listen.
6. Memory improves.
7. We learn to be a better self through listening.

There are basically four types of listening. Most people practice or more accurately do not practice what is called, inactive listening.

Inactive listening is inefficient and unproductive. It is the type of listening that we all get mad at. When someone tells us they are listening but they look like they are somewhere else.

Then there is selective listening. We hear only what we want to hear showing little concern for what the other person needs for us to hear.

Active Listening is a conscious effort to hear not only the words but listen for the message being sent by the speaker. Active listening takes into account the intent of the speaker and the body language. Active listening attempts to be nonjudgemental.

Reflective listening. Is very much like active listening. We listen to the whole message. We use reflective listening to resolve a conflict or a problem.

Inactive and selective listening is demonstrated all around us. For the purpose of learning more accurate communication we will discuss active and reflective listening. Both of which are summed up in the phrase active listening.

Active listening listens to intent, assesses the speaker's nonverbal communication, controls our nonverbal communication, and empathetically and nonjudgmentally listens.

Listening to the intent of the speaker means we are listening as to why things are said rather than to putting all the importance on what is said. The better we know the person the easier and more accurate we listen with intent.

Nonverbal communication is often called body language and tone of voice. Verbal communication deals only with the words spoken but not how they are spoken. It has been said that 93% of our communication is nonverbal. Of that 55% is body language and 35% is the tone of voice that is used.

Monitoring our own nonverbals means that we do our best to hear what is being said but not through our biases. We attempt to put our preconceived ideas aside to hear what is really going on.

Listening with empathy and not being judgmental lets the speaker know we care about them. We accept him even if his ideas are different. We convey the thought that we are willing to hear him out.

In order to do the above we need to evaluate our listening skills.

Rate each answer 1-5 1=never, 2,3,4=Sometimes, 5 = always

EVALUATING YOUR LISTENING SKILLS

Do you think you understood what was said only to find yourself asking what did they mean when they said.....

Do you find it hard to concentrate on what someone is saying because of distractions such as noise or movement?

Are you distracted because of internal things like, worry, fear, being ill prepared or daydreaming.

Do you find yourself responding to what the speaker implies rather that listening to what is being said?

Do you respond with angry words, stated or inferred, that for all logical purposes should not provoke your anger?

Do you have trouble reading body language?

Is it difficult to be nonjudgmental when we do not agree?

Are you preparing your response while they are yet speaking?

Do you listen selectively, hearing only the words or ideas you want to hear?

Do certain words, phrases or actions trigger certain positive or negative responses in you?

Do you find yourself saying, "What did you say?" even though you heard the words?

Do you depend on others to interpret what happened at your meeting?

13-20---very good listener
21-32---fairly good listener
33-45---average listener
46-58---fairly poor listener
59-65---poor listener

How did you do? Would you like to communicate better?

TIPS TO COMMUNICATE BETTER

1. sit or stand where you can maintain eye contact.
2. sit or stand where you can read body language.
3. remove sunglasses.
4. eliminate outside distractions as much as possible
5. eliminate as many internal distractions as possible. Attempt to free your mind of previous thoughts.

ACTIVE LISTENING

1. listen to the other person
2. repeat back to them what you think you heard, paraphrase.
3. allow them to say," yes that's right," or, "no what I meant was..."
4. if they correct what you paraphrased to them say, "Oh, I see you meant.....again paraphrase.
5. allow them to respond. This goes back and forth until both have a clear understanding of what was really said.
6. now it is time to talk resolutions.

I consider the first five steps in active listening to be the first half and step six to be the second half of active listening. To better describe the second half we could say, now that we each understand what the other person wants and feels and why this situation is hurting them we can come to a resolution. Then we;

1. make a suggestion of what we think will help with this problem.
2. listen to what the other person thinks about the suggestion.
3. They paraphrase back what they heard you say then they add how they feel

about it. They say, "what I hear you saying is that you are happy with going to New York for our vacation. I don't want to go because I haven't been feeling well."

4. first person validates their feedback and suggest perhaps another solution. "Okay I understand you don't want to go to New York because you are not feeling well. I think you need to call the doctor. Get a checkup. See if you feel better then we will decide if we go to New York.

5. next person; "That is a good idea. But what I would like is to get a checkup. But I would really rather wait until September to go rather than now."

This process goes back and forth with feedback, information from both parties until a compromise is made that both parties are comfortable living with.

My husband and I worked the first half of active listening for five years before we knew how to work step six. We would talk about how we felt. Paraphrase back to each other what we heard. And apologize to each other for any pain caused to the other. After I began to learn more about being functional and exactly what it is I began to say, "No, this isn't it. We need not to stop at apologizing. I want to work out a solution we can live with if at all possible. This I think will make life run smoother in the future." We had many rough moments. I'm sure you will too. I can also reassure you that we get out of recovery what we are willing to put into it. Work and pain I am not afraid of. What I do strongly distaste was the misery of dysfunction. Pain is a part of life. Much pain can be reduced when we communicate effectively. We can have pain and still know we are loved. We can be functional and not be happy. However functional knows that I will do what I need to do, I will do what I can do about the things I can change. Functional knows that we will not stay stuck in this pain, even though we may feel like it. Functional knows we can work it out, sort our feelings, talk to people who care, write about it, think about it, ask for help from whoever we think is most appropriate for what we are dealing with. Functional knows that life goes on and we are normal people, with normal problems. Functional knows that communication is the key to solutions. Functional gives that same gift to our children.

DYSFUNCTIONAL CONVERSATION

Your teenager says, "I hate school. There's too much homework. The teachers never listen or try to be fair. Then I have my job. I don't get to do anything."

The dysfunctional parent says, "I had to do it and so do you. Quit complaining about your lot in life. You're not going to lay around here. Life is not fair and you just have to accept that."

FUNCTIONAL CONVERSATION

Your teenager says, "I hate school. There's too much homework. The teachers never listen or try to be fair. Then I have my job. I don't get to do anything."

Functional Parent says: I get the impression you are feeling pressured?"

Teenager: Yeah, it's just too much.
Parent: We all feel like that at times. What would you like to do to take off some of the pressure you feel now?"
Teenager: I'd like to make those teachers be fair to us, as students."
Parent: Can you think of a way to do that?
Teenager: No, it will never happen.
Parent: I think you're probably right. What else could help you out with your schedule right now?
Teenager: I've been thinking about asking for fewer hours at work, or maybe a week off.
Parent: I think that's a good idea.

What would any of us have given for the type of respect shown to this teenager? Growing up means accepting life is not fair. Growing up means being allowed to make some decisions on our own. Growing up means we would like to make decisions on our own and still have the security of knowing our loving parents are there to guide us and love us.

What was communicated by the parent in the above conversation? The parent offered no solutions. What the parent did do was;

1. The father listened to the feelings of his son. The teenager knew it because his father paraphrased back to him the feelings he heard in his son's words.

2. The father did not imply that his son was incompetent in some way because he was not able to keep up with his schedule.

3. The father let his son know this is normal it happens to everyone.

4. The father showed respect for the age, feelings, and intelligence his son possesses by asking him what he wanted to do.

5. When the son suggested a solution the father complimented him on his idea.

All of the above constitutes function. The less biases we have the better able we are to give to our children the above. The more biases or dysfunction we have the more difficult it will be for us to give this gift to ourselves as well as to them. things that get in the way of our listening judgmental and bringing us closer to the dysfunction conversation above are sometimes called filters. My filters are;

1. my expectations of the speaker or situation.
2. my relationship with this person, co workers, my spouse.
3. my present personal situation
4. my emotions prior to this communication situation.

Taking a look at each of these aspects helps us to understand how they apply. Our expectations, we expect such and such from this business or personal conversation but it or they did not live up to our expectations. We were expecting to hear one thing and we hear something else instead. In our sample conversation consider that the father is quit proud of his son's ability to work a job and keep a high grade point average. Is he expecting to hear his son complain how he hates school?

He might be in a original state of shock. If he is not careful he may overreact to his son's statement. If he had assumed he knew what his son was going to say, assuming all is well and wonderful he may come away from the conversation disappointed in his son.

Part of our expectations have to do with the speaker. As when we must listen to a business lecture or meeting we conclude, Oh, no he's boring. Or she'll lecture me. So and so is overbearing. Our jump to conclusions before the conversation can and will stifle our conversations with that person.

We can however control our expectation. Several things that help in this direction are to sit quietly ahead of time and thing about a personal conversation. Write down what we expect about our topic, situation or speaker. We will then become aware of what are barriers to listening are. A large part of active listening is to listen without judging what they say through our preconceived ideas.

We also can test our reactions. See how we respond to certain ideas. Ask yourself, "How will I respond if they say..." Use this technique in situations where you have difficulty communicating or hearing information you do not like. (selective listening)

My existing relationship with the person I need to listen to- The more we dislike a person the harder it is to listen objectively. the more we like a person, the harder it is to actively listen objectively. The relationship colors the communication. Set aside feelings and listen objectively.

My current personal situation is reflected in my ability to listen. If I am unemployed, experiencing a divorce or other negative things I will look through my experience in that light. If my personal life is happy the same is true. If my personal life is inhibiting my ability to listen I can;

1. distance myself mentally or physically from my personal life.

2. when commuting, use this time to leave personal problems at home.

3. practice self talk--I empower myself to be my best today by leaving personal problems at home.

4. share my concerns with someone who is a good listener and can keep a confidence.

5. make a list of my personal concerns or keep a journal. Writing out problems gives clarity to any situation.

6. if chronic personal problems make doing these things extremely difficult, seek counseling.

My mindset immediately before a conversation with anyone affects and effects my listening ability. We may find it difficult to concentrate because we are angry about something that just happened. When in the mid of conversation and the phone rings, stop the conversation then;

1. let the phone ring several times

2. create a cool down buffer zone if possible. Spend a few minutes sorting mail or some other trifle thing. This allows me to detach from negative emotions before interacting with others.

3. exercise if possible. Go for a walk.. Go to the rest room. Take a break.

4. breathing in slow and slowly let it out. Breath in - feel the feelings. Breath out very slow-let out all the anxiety that accompanied those feelings. Do at least ten times. Now we can be more objective in the next conversation.

Dysfunction is when we take out our bad pent up feelings from one situation out or other people in another conversation. Any of the above techniques help to lessen our tension.

The above information is dealing with what is referred to as I messages. We listen then we express what we heard others say and how we feel by saying,

What I heard you saying is,

I think you feel pressured.

How I see this situation is.

I think we need to talk.

I understand that my attitudes make it harder for me to listen objectively.

I can work on my communication skills.

FEELING MESSAGES

Sometimes more will be required to communicate to the other person that you have listened and understood them then the use of I statement. In addition to I statements we can add Feeling Statements. When we express feeling statements we are allowing them to have their feelings. I can paraphrase to them not what they said but what I heard they feel.

For example your daughter comes home feeling rejected because her coach showed her friend a list of those who made track finals and she is not on it. She say, "I just know he doesn't like me because if he liked me he would not want to embarrass me by telling my best friend I did not make the finals.

As a parent I want to jump in and fix it for her. But the best thing I can do for her is to let her have her feelings even if it is grief. My empathic feelings message can be, "You feel rejected an hurt because you feel he was inconsiderate. You feel hurt because you feel embarrassed. You feel that Mr. Johnson doesn't like you because he did an inconsiderate thing."

ACTIVE I MESSAGES

In the first type of I message I let the other person know I understand. The words I understand by themselves are not sufficient. I understand that you..... lets the person hear back what they stated. They know they were understood. Learning active listening was the light of my life. No longer need I say something, wonder if they understand, say something else, hope they understand, ask them if they understand, they say they do. I'm not sure. At a later time when some plans are confused they say, "You said..." I say, "That's not what I said at all. I said....." Active listen eliminates all the confusion as well as lets it's participates know they were understood. Now I say what is on my mind as bottom line as possible, unless I am talking through some heavy emotions to a person with whom I trust in their confidence. I feel listened too. I feel heard. If that person does not know active listening we can choose to teach them if we feel they are receptive. Several people of thanked me saying it has ended much of their frustration with others in their life.

Now we know how to use I messages and feeling messages. The active I message is also important. It works like this. When your daughter comes home with her feelings about Mr. Johnson her track teacher you can use an I message to paraphrase to her what you hear. She feels Mr. Johnson does not like her. You can say, "When you talk about Mr. Johnson not liking you I can't help but be concerned because I think your decision is based on one incident. I think it might be a good idea to get more information before coming to such a drastic decision."

Here I am giving off, I messages." I am not insulting my daughter's opinion. She can think what she likes. I can think what I like. This leaves the door open for her to express her opinions to me. At the same time, I am offering the loving hand of parental guidance (feedback).

In our example of the son who says, "I think I will ask for a cut in hours or a week off." I, the parent, could say, "that's a possible solution. I also think it would be a good idea to see if you could arrange to get a study hall put into your schedule at school. What do you think?"

Ask opened ended questions. Questions that have no right or wrong answer. Never insult the answer. Our response is best accepted if we react to the idea. "Well I can see why you think so but I don't feel this idea will work in this situation." It does not become a rejecting of the person. Because you do not like an idea does not mean you do not value him or her.

Respond in the present, not the past. "You're always late." "You're always saying," If this is our response we are no longer being nonjudgemental. A nonjudgemental approach would say, "When you are late, I feel that the others are cheated because we have to wait for you." or "I hate being late. I don't want to miss the beginning of the movie."

We can also help to break the cycle of dysfunction by responding by describing a thing not by evaluation it. Don't say, "You're just blowing this whole thing out of proportion." Say, "I hear you saying your name was not on the track team list." Now you can ask open ended questions.

To communicate effectively means to listen empathetically and nonjudgmentally. This can only be accomplished by putting aside our biases, our mental blocks or as some refer to them as our filters. We filter what we hear through what we already believe. Recovery is about learning what we believe, being willing to change the beliefs we had that have come to be to our disadvantage, holding strong convictions to guide our moral standard, and still being able to listen to others without feeling that must hold the same standards as we.

Our filters or mental blocks are the core of what we are as a person. This is my real self speaking and listening. These are beliefs about our values, our religious upbringing, our culture, the region we grew up in, and our parents political party. If and when our buttons are pushed and we do not know why we may need to ask ourselves:

Does this person remind you of someone from your past? His voice, body language, looks, word choice. What emotional response is going on with you?

Does the situation you are reacting to remind you of a similar incident in the past?

Is my reaction a result of some conflict, whether it is personal, religious, political or philosophical? What is that conflict?

Is my emotional reaction recycled by a prejudice of bias?

We are starting to understand ourselves, other people and the world of communication. Communication is the link between our true self and the rest of the world. When we have accurate communication and know how to use it in everyday situations we are becoming functional. Recently I read that it is better to seek to understand rather than to be understood. This I feel is accurate. This is not the dysfunction of caring more about others than myself but the function of connecting with the rest of the universe. Here again is a paradox of recovery. When I seek to be understood chances are-I don't receive it. When I seek to understand others chances are -I receive understanding. When I understand others I will be understood to a greater degree. What will be understood about myself is whatever is my degree of empathy, love, and genuine caring. What will be understood about me is my level of love for my God and my fellow man.

In short seeking to understand others is a form of spirituality. A high level of maturity. While seeking to be understood could be compared to striving after the wind.

Accurate communication brings understanding of others. Since I understand others, why my family was dysfunctional, I have been able to release the shame I carried over many years. I have been able to feel loved, secure, worthy, competent, self respecting, and growing, ever growing. All the above add up to joy of heart. When I have joy of heart I have love, joy, kindness, goodness, mildness, faith, long suffering, and self control. All fruitages of God's spirit. How could I not feel loved and understood.

THINGS TO KNOW ABOUT UNDERSTANDING

1. When we say to others I'm trying to understand we need to look at ourselves and see what is getting in the way of our understanding.
2. We can understand intellectually and not understand empathetically.
3. We can understand empathetically and not agree.
4. Understanding does not mean we approve or agree.
5. When I say I 'm trying to understand I am saying I am trying to see your viewpoint. It does not mean that I am trying to come around to your way of thinking.
6. We can say this because surely we can find something even if it is a grain of sand in what they say that we agree with or understand.
7. Active listening helps the other person to express their concerns.
8. When I find myself becoming judgmental, not understanding, not wanting to understand, I can FLOAT WITH IT. I will strive to relax my shoulders breath slow, release tension my my body and attempt to listen. I can ask for God's help.

Active listening is about breaking the cycle of dysfunction. It is about learning to release our controlling child and allowing our natural child the true me to say, "Hello world I'm glad I'm here. I'm happy to meet you. I care not only about my feelings. I care about yours. I will listen to you like I want you to listen to me."

Active Listening is about breaking the cycle of control. If I tell you this loud enough and long enough you will get this through your thick head. Active listening is showing our caring for other people. We listen to why they feel without judging why they feel. We are attempting to see their heart, their core, their true self. When we are able to practice active listening we are able to break our cycle of dysfunction and give them a taste to see the goodness of recovery. We cannot know it may be the first time some one genuinely listened to them. It may be the first time they felt listened to. Can we reach down into our core and give to ourselves and another the precious gift of ending the cycle of act, react, react some more? Are we by using active listening saying in effect, "I care. I care about you and your problems. I will allow you the dignity of feeling what you need to feel even if I don't like what you feel. Even if you don't like what you feel. I will listen to you. I will not try to solve your problems but I will show you by listening to you that I have confidence in your ability to solve your problems. If then you would like suggestions (feedback) I can offer the same without feeling you must do as I suggested for you to be handling this situation correctly. I will let you empower yourself by respecting your decision to handle this situation as you need to to take care of your needs. Not the needs I feel you should have. I will be happy for your personal growth, even when such grow has to come your way through pain and trouble. I will not be happy about your pain but we will both understand that pain is a part of life and by feeling it not by shutting it off or pretending it's less than it is we learn that we have abilities beyond what we knew. We become more and more functional knowing we can handle this situation and other difficult situations that will come our way in our lifetime. We are aware that our self respect is being built one brick at a time."

With the above rhetorical I would like to say that we have broken the cycle of dysfunction.

REVIEW TO LISTENING EFFECTIVELY SKILLS

Listen with empathy.

Listen nonjudgmentally.

Speak in I messages showing you understand.

Express feeling messages to help the other to be able to say what they need to say.

Use active I messages.

Ask open ended questions.

Respond to the behavior or idea not the person.

Respond in the present tense.

Respond by describing, not evaluating.

Respond nonjudgmentally.

Don't force someone to share their feelings.

Use reflective listening to highlight important issues.

Respond as accurately as you can.

Respond as honestly as you can.

Reflect back positive and pleasant feelings.

Don't expect to get active listening perfect.

If the problem is to big for both of you seek expert advice.

Now we are aware of the skills involved in communication. Communication does not start with how to talk. It starts with how to listen. Almost everyone is aware their listening are not what they would like them to be. Herein we will discuss five things we can do to instantly improve our listening abilities. They are;

1. Use our thinking ability

2. Listen for the complete message. What is said verbally and what is not said but is shown by body language and tone of voice.

3. Whenever possible eliminate outside and internal distractions.

4. Stay motivated. Take the initial step in the conversation to be a good listener.

5. Use both active listening and reflective listening.

Using our thinking ability when listening involves these skills;

1. We listen for accuracy. Listen to the facts and the specifics.

2. Listen to their words and their ideas. Listen like we have never heard this information.

3. Listen for inconsistencies. This keeps us mentally alert.

4. Write "listen with my mind" in a place where I can see it each day.

5. If I am reacting emotionally I need to do a awareness check. Ask myself, What can I do to listen to this person objectively?"

Listening for the whole message verbal and nonverbal involves;

1. Think about their choice of words. If a person says they went home the inflection is entirely different than if they say, "I went back to the house."

2. Maintain eye contact. This lets the other person know you are listening.

3. Watch for body language. Much is automatic.

4. Watch facial expressions.

5. Listen to their tone of voice.

6. Respond to what we think they are saying. Now listen closely to their response to us.

Eliminating outside and inside distractions involves;[2]

1. Radio and stereo for serious conversations.

2. Move to a different room, close the door or whatever is necessary to have as much quite as possible.

3. Go into a listening situation with our mind as open as possible. Detach from internal concerns, fear, worry, and anger. Write them down of a piece of paper and deal with them later.

4. If this environment cannot be controlled to the extent to allow decent communication do not be afraid to say, "could we move this conversation to...." or "I think it would be a good idea to do this later. When is a good time for you?"

5. Try to pick neutral ground for the both of us. Whoever is on home turf has the advantage.

Staying motivated to listen involves:

1. Each week pick out a skill. Make it a weekly goal. Write it down and put it on your bathroom mirror. Here you can see it every morning as you ready for your day.

2. Make a list of what I want to accomplish this week by using active listening.

3. After the first week make a list of what you have accomplished. This is allowing ourself to receive credit for what we have done and will empower us to keep up the good work.

4. Set a goal to pass your new knowledge on to someone else. This may be a person with whom you wish to build better communication. As both of you strive to put communication skills into practice you will be sometimes frustrated and many times

delighted. But either way you will be breaking the cycle of dysfunction. Communication is the opposite of dysfunction.

Use active and reflective listening, both use the same principles but their purpose is different. Reflective listening lets the other person know how they look and that you understand what they have said. Active listening uses I statement and adds what you think and feel about what they express.

Choose which is the most appropriate for this situation. Reflective listening is for one on one conversations. The speaker is wrestling with a problem and needs a listener, not advice. He just needed someone to talk to. Active listening is used in group problem solving situations or when one on one want feedback.

We will need to realize that reflective listening takes time. We will develop these skills over a period of weeks or several months even when we are concentrating on the development of these skills. We are learning to listen with empathy and not to judge. This shows we care. It allows the other person to think out loud without being afraid of how you will evaluate him or her.

Next comes the most commonly asked question; What if I do all this and they don't, will it work? Does all this do any good? My answer has to be, yes it does. Of course some will not appreciate our listening skills. Some may feel intimidated. Here we tie back into their dysfunction. I do not, I will not take the blame for any of their misperceptions. I will speak as accurate and as honest as I know how. I will not deliberately leave a wrong impression. If from there another person resents it when I paraphrase their thought back to them I can remind myself that I am communicating in a way that is most effective and most people respond to well. In all the time that I have used active listening, about seven years, I have only come across two people that were upset when what they said was paraphrased back to them. This speaks of their insecurities not my communication abilities.

Others may be poor listeners. They may wish to know more about how to listen more effectively. By using our listening skills we can help poor listeners to understand what we are saying. We do so by teaching others active and reflective listening. We will always find some who admire our listening ability. You can then say, "Something that helped me was learning not to judge when others speak." or "Something that helped me a lot was learning how to listen when they speak instead of planning my response when they speak. When I was planning responses while they spoke I could not listen to the best of my ability." We can use our conversations with friends and acquaintances to pass on tidbits of information. If they show much interest you can tell them about a good book you read or a class you took that helped you learn to listen and communicate more effectively. We can also explain that active listening solves many problems. When I repeat back to you what I think I heard, you are free to say, "Yes," and feel the joy of knowing you were understood. On the other hand if there is a misunderstanding we can correct this problem now before it causes another problem down the line. How do we know if they want more information?

When someone compliments your listening skills suggest ways they can learn more about how to listen. If we have just attended a seminar, tell co-workers or family, ask them to help you in you efforts to put this into practice. When someone asks how you learned to listen well, tell them. When a group you must work with is frustrated and beset with problems because of poor listening skills, tell them there is a way to eliminate many of the frustrations going on here. Then explain.

We can aid others in their search for better listening skills by sending nonverbal messages to those who are not receptive to learning about effective listening and the skills involved. We can send a message to let them know they are not listening. Some of these nonverbal ways to communicate to them they're not listening would be;

1. look puzzled when they respond. Let your expression show you do not understand how they got that out of what you said.

2. frown, if disapproving of how they responded because they did not hear you. This is not judging their ideas. It is a response to their inactive or selective listening.

3. in a business setting take notes on their response. This will let them know they will be accountable for what they said.

4. move forward to show you are listening, use facial expressions showing you don't understand why they responded the way they did.

5. lean back in your chair looking like "I am thinking about what you just said to

me." pose. Then respond verbally and discuss how they didn't accurately listen to what you were saying.

An important element to remember is they do not know how to listen because of their dysfunction. In their dysfunction they may also ignore or misinterpret your cues. This is their responsibility. You can only do what you can do.

Another effective way to help a poor listener is to ask questions to make them think. These may be open ended or closed questions. Open ended questions are general in nature and focus on issues that the listener hasn't heard. They need to be phrased in such a way that they lead the listener to think about what you said that you feel they did not hear.

Closed questions are specific in nature. They question the listener about what you just said. Open ended questions can be used in almost any situation Closed questions can be taken as assertive, combative, or aggressive. Use them carefully. Closed ended questions indicate control. Better used by an employer than an employee. A parent not a child. A police officer not the person getting the ticket.

We can use reflective listening to keep a poor listener on track. To a poor listener we can say,

"I hear you saying... Did you hear me saying...?"

"I understand your point." then explain the point letting him know you really do understand. Proceed with "I wonder if you understood my point, then explain your point."

"Let's look at what you said in comparison to what I said."

Say, "I wonder if you understand what I said. I do not get that impression. Then repeat your thought.

In this way we are showing them a good role model of effective listening and conversation. With those we know well our spouse, child, friend, long time co-worker, or perhaps a parent we can work with what we know are their emotional and mental filters, blocks. We can phrase what we have to say so their filters will work for us not against us. Appeal to the need in them. This anticipates arguments and concerns on their part. We can make a list of what we think they do not want to hear. We do not do this to control the situation. We do not do this to manipulate their response. We do this so that we are able to express to them what we feel needs to be expressed and give to them the opportunity of hearing information that can be helpful to them if they allow it. We do this so we can learn to be effective and communicative. We have learned in the process of breaking our cycle of dysfunction that we have the right to express our needs. Yes we do. But I do not believe that it is the same as expressing our needs by cutting the other person off at the knees. Being functional means that we express our needs while still considering the feelings of others. If we know they feel strongly about... we would out of consideration and considering chances of their hearing our side without being combative are greatly enhanced by stating our feelings and needs in a way that does not insult their feelings. We are in effect making what we have to say palatable. In doing so we can mirror their nonverbals such as body language, tone of voice, or pace of speech. Be careful as to the where and when's with this practice. Don't overdo it. Most of all we will avoid being combative. If we become combative we have not demonstrated the art of communication. They will have missed the point. If we feel we may become combative remember it takes one to start the fight and two or more to keep it going. Count to ten and breath slowly. Ask yourself, "what is the issue we are discussing?" We are endeavoring to stick to the issue. If this is not possible to do with both of you in a relatively calm state say, "Can we discuss this later today or tomorrow? When is good for you?"

We have endeavored to use our nonverbals to another to illustrate to another more effective communication. Another important aspect of using nonverbals for better communication is to monitor our nonverbals. When we are able to do so the other person will feel freer to communicate to us. If we are in agreement with the speaker we ten to mirror his body language. This allows them to know you understand. Whether or not the other person knows about active listening they will mirror you and put them in the mode for active listening.

We can now use our body language to show we are listening. We can:

1. sit up in the chair
2. lean forward.

3. cup chin in hand showing we are thoughtfully listening.
4. nod our head in agreement.

Facial expressions while important are easy to fake. Make facial expressions equal to our other nonverbal cues. We say we love an idea with a frown on our face we are sending a double message. Which one is correct? Usually it is the body language that gives the real clue. If I smile and cross my arms this too is conflicting signals. Crossed arms equal I don't agree or stay away.

If you disagree we are not left without choices. We can reflect our disagreement. We can choose to look neutral. Showing our disagreement is acceptable as long as it does not start a conflict. A neutral face shows you are being nonjudgmental.

If we agree with the speaker smile. Put I don't understand what you are saying look on your face if you are confused. In any and all cases use eye contact as much as possible. Use gestures. Gestures show you are listening. Posture and upper body moves are included in our gestures. Here are some indications of the messages we send to others with our body language.

When we sit or stand straight it shows we are listening.

Crossed arms and legs give the impression you are closed. You disagree, feel trapped or stubborn.

Restless movements signals boredom.

Nervous gestures such as tapping a pen bouncing our leg up and down show we are bored or nervous.

When we mirror the speaker's body language we are showing we agree.

The biggest cause for the breakup of marriages is that people feel they are not listened to. Stable relationships are built on good listening. Here we put active listening into effect by listening with empathy and nonjudgemental. We show we are doing this by:

1. Putting aside what we are doing when our spouse talks.

2. Listening with our whole body. Maintain eye contact. Move forward. These are I am listening to you messages.

3. Controlling our emotions. Do not react to our hot buttons.

4. If our spouse is upset use reflective listening to help him or her work through the problem. Your mate may not want you to solve their problem. They may just want you to listen. Provide emotional support by listening. Do not try to fix. Show them you have confidence in their ability to find their own solutions.

5. Listen the way you would want them to listen to you.

This is probably the longest chapter in this book. Accurate communication is the crux of breaking the cycle of dysfunction. We break the cycle when we learn new more effective skills and teach our children the same skills. A friend of mine who grew up in the most functional family I know does most of these things without knowing there is a vocabulary for it. When I talk about it she says, "That's it. That's what it's called." These processes are so automatic to her that she and her family do them without a thought. This is because they were taught what I refer to as the preferable pedagogy.

We teach our children how to be good communicators by teaching them to be good nonjudgmental listeners. Teaching our children to be good listeners involves;

1. Role modeling good listening behavior. This includes all of the skills in this chapter. Communication is what I longed for my entire life. I have found it. I cherish it. I attempt to model it for my family and friends. I do feel great joy over knowing the things I have modeled have started others on the road of recovery and the path to breaking the cycle of dysfunction.

2. Teaching my children to be consistent. This I do by being consistent myself. Dysfunction makes promises to children and then finds a way not to uphold those promises by saying, "If you kids hadn't of..... I would do it. But you blew it." The child may have made a mistake. This however does not mean the parent has the right to be inconsistent. Functional parents withhold a privilege if that was part of the original

plan. If you be quite during my visit with Susie I will take you for ice cream. If the child is quite we uphold our end of the bargain. Many dysfunctional parents will say after the visit, "Yes, you were quite but I didn't like the way you looked at her." The parent is inconsistent and the child does not know what to expect. The child learns not to listen to what we have said.

3. We teach our children to read body language by saying what you see. Something like, "see how she leaned forward to listen close." We can also teach them the accurate meaning of facial gestures. Recently I saw a flyer with many faces upon it. Probably twenty to thirty. These were of the happy face type however, they were not all happy faces. They were feeling faces. The feelings expressed were happy, sad, angry, grief, smug, arrogant, worried, bored and many others. To be functional, to listen effectively, to understand body language effectively, we must also learn to read the most common gesture of all, facial gestures. In dysfunction feelings are labeled wrongly. We are then confused about what we see. When my three year old grandson was upset he made up his little face. I said, "You look sad." He said, "No, I'm mad." "That face looks sad to me." Sometimes it is the other way around. But understanding our feelings is crucial to having them labeled correctly as a child. If we were nervous and got yelled at for being angry then when ever we are nervous or having anxiety we think we are dealing with out of control anger.

By accurately identifying facial gestures we teach our children accurate communication and good listening skills. When another person is nervous our children will not be afraid of the other person anger. They will know this person is nervous. All these skills are vital in breaking the cycle of dysfunction.

4. Listen to our children with empathy and they will probably do it for others.

5. Discuss with our children their responses when you feel they are being judgmental. This will teach them to be less judgmental. In the illustration earlier in the chapter about the daughter who felt the teacher did not like her because he showed a list of track team members to her friend we see a mother appropriately pointing out to the daughter a point to consider. Her words were, "when you talk about Mr. Johnson

not liking you I can't help but be concerned because I think your decision is based on one incident. I think it might be a good idea to get more information before coming to such a drastic decision. "

Her mother did not chastise her daughter. She did give to her daughter the gift of saying, "here is something I would like you to think about. Maybe you need to open your mind and reconsider." A precious gift from a functional mother. One who at no time invalidated her daughter's feelings by saying, "that's ridiculous." Another style of dysfunction would have sided entirely with the daughter in a statement like, "How dare he. I can see how you would be upset. What made him think he had the right to do that. I will see to it he losses his job. What an idiot. If he thinks he's going to get by with this." This allows the mother to feel needed by fixing the daughter's problem. She also feels some sense of satisfaction in being able to release some of her anger at an authority figure. Sadly enough though no one in this situation will grow or mature to a healthy functional adult.

6. We can also watch television with our children. Talk about what people are saying with their words and their body signals. We can also discuss how the people in the situation handle their conflicts.

Accurate communication is based in good effective listening skills. Under normal smooth flowing circumstances we can say, I want, I need , and I feel. But how is our communication affected and effected in times of conflict. This is the true test of our communication abilities. Verbal judo and accurate communication styles will allow us to fight fair.

END OF SECTION TWO

FIGHTING WITH DIGNITY

Dysfunction is in essence the inability to handle conflict in an appropriate manner. We feared conflict due to our myths about anger. Some fear if they make another person mad or angry that person will leave them. Another reaction to anger is, people don't leave because they are angry. They may stay around and beat you up but people just don't leave because they get angry. They may leave if they allow anger to build up over a period of time. Both responses cause the same dreadful end: either I must be nice. I must not say what I need, I must not express my anger or vent, dominate, and control. Or I can show my anger to keep others at a distance. No one will dare conflict with me. Both reactions are a result of fear of what may happen to us in the event someone dares to conflict with us.

What has been learned in only recent years is: it is not how many times we conflict with another that makes or breaks a relationship but how conflict is handled when it occurs that makes or breaks this relationship. We need not fear our anger or theirs when it is handled appropriately. This could better be called fighting with dignity.

The easiest way to act appropriately with our anger is to overcome what is called outerdirected. Outerdirected is when we let things outside of ourselves control our self esteem. Things outside of ourself will control our moods. If I lose a friend in life or death I will be sad. If I am accused falsely I will be mad. These are the normal emotions of life. Being outerdirected adds to this pain the pain of, "I'm not good enough because I am sad or mad," or whatever emotion we feel. If I feel I am not able to get this right because of the things that happen this is outerdirected. Outerdirected is dysfunction. Functional is innerdirected. I can be sad, mad, happy, fearful or feel any emotion I need to feel without it reflecting on my value as a person.

There is no faster way for us to get angry then when someone says something that taps directly into what is for us a self esteem issue. This is why dysfunction sets us up for conflict. We then attempt to avoid conflict. Result: stress, stress, and more stress. Dysfunction is all about lack of self esteem.

We can learn many effective ways to handle anger appropriately. Some of them are:

1. learn active listening skills
2. learn fight fair rules
3. learn verbal judo

I believe before we can learn the above three skills we must take a look at ourselves. We must begin to understand our dysfunction. We can look at the situations that occur when we get angry. Analyze them for:

1. what is a common factor in each of these situations. At first we may not see there is something or anything similar in any of the situations. This leads to step two.

2. If there is no similarity in the incidents themselves stop to think of the first feeling you are aware of seconds before the surge of anger.

It could be;

a. they must think I'm stupid
b. they are doing this to me again.
c. I don't fit in here.
d. I better not say that.

Once we identify with the feeling that produces our anger we can begin to work on the issue and how it connects to our self esteem. We will delightfully find there are not a lot of things over which we get angry. Every time I state this to a class the first reaction I get is, "There isn't?" "There Isn't," is always my reply. There will be several principles that mean a lot to us. When we feel they have been violated this triggers our anger.

How we handle conflict may well be dependent on the reason for our conflict. Consider two types of conflict. First there is conflict for the sake of conflict, we normally call this venting our feelings on others, being aggressive. Then there is constructive conflict. Conflict we can use to learn about ourselves, about others, about our and their problem solving abilities. With constructive conflict comes some type of resolution. This does not indicate conflict will always work out the way we prefer. Quoting from Profile of Abuse,

I can say, 'I want, I need, or I feel, but just because I say I want, I need, or I feel does not mean that I expect to get everything I want, I need, or I feel." This is called maturity. It does however make us feel better knowing that someone cares enough to listen with understanding to what my wants and needs and feelings are. This greatly lessens my stress and my potential for conflict.

We are not discussing how to go about not having conflict. The title of this chapter is fighting with dignity. We are talking about how to handle conflict when it does arise even though we would prefer it not to arise. Everyone has conflict in their life. Dysfunction had taught me to feel like a failure whenever conflict arose. Today I have accepted functional means conflict need not ruin my day, my week, or my life. I am not a failure because I have conflict. I am not lacking kindness and caring for others because I have anger. What I am lacking is the ability to hide from my right to say, "Stop, I cannot allow you to talk to me in that tone of voice." I accept my conflicts with no guilt, no depression, no I'm not good enough to get this right. And best of all with the point of view that I handle most conflicts appropriately and I have grown as a person and have peace of mind and contentment I did not have while dysfunctional. Each of these growth steps has been due to things I learned through conflict.

What a happy day it was when I could say, "We sit at the kitchen table and fight our way through some solutions." We fight with dignity. We talk, sometimes through our teeth. We sit at the table, not running around the house, walking out on each other. I can be angry at you and have the sense of dignity to sit at this table and tell you the reasons why. When I am able to do such I grow.

I GROW BECAUSE

1. I can feel good about myself for any degree of improvement I made in how I handled this conflict.

2. I feel good that I need not run from this conflict to stay calm.

3. I feel good that I am not afraid of being injured in this conflict.

4. I feel good knowing I have no fear of what I might do to others in my anger.

5. I know I can handle this anger in a more constructive way.

6. I improve my self esteem because I can give myself a pat on the back for a job well done.

7. I increase my confidence level in myself in other areas of life. If I can improve in this very difficult area I can improve in other ways too.

8. I can now handle other feelings in a more appropriate way.

9. With my increased confidence level comes ever increasing self esteem. Now we are treating the real issue.

TO REMEMBER

The better my self esteem the more I will act appropriately in difficult situations.

DIFFERENCES BETWEEN DESTRUCTIVE AND CONSTRUCTIVE CONFLICT.

The Chinese have two different symbols used together for the word conflict. One means danger. The other means opportunity. This is aptly so as we will see in this discussion of both types of conflict. Two types of conflict are:

1. interpersonal = a disagreement in a situation within a relationship.
2. intrapersonal = inside ourself.

The relationship is the key. The quality of the relationship makes it an opportunity or a dangerous conflict. We now work on the relationship.

Anger results when we feel threatened, frustrated, irritated, or uncomfortable.

The bottom line is: we are afraid of what is going to happen to me. Our needs are not being met. When we understand ourselves better we are in a position to make better choices.

A constructive conflict is when all parties work together to solve a problem. Some benefits of a constructive conflict are:

1. parties involved come to understand each other better.
2. constructive conflict lessens future potential for arguments.
3. parties are likely to feel good about decisions they have come to.
4. all parties will feel good about each other if they feel good about their mutual resolution. One where everyone gets something they want.

Our conflict is much more likely to be a constructive conflict when we first ask the following questions of ourselves.

1. What conflicts in the past are we bringing into this situation? These will make the present situation harder to cope with effectively. We now have the weight of past conflicts as well as the present conflict. How I once put it, "I cannot fight on two

battlefronts at one time." True and accurate. "I think if I settle the things of the past I'll handle the things going on now better." In our effort to control both our feelings about the past and the feelings we have about the present we become easily overwhelmed. We are afraid of losing control, our right to have a measure of control or say so in this issue. If the past event similar to this event took power, control, personal rights, and self esteem from us we fear this situation will do the same. This intensifies the anger of the present. Leaving us little dignity, little ability to fight with dignity.

2. What is our level of commitment? Do we feel valued? We fear it will always be like this, always has. We are not living in the now. Taking care of the problem of the moment without dragging in past events and feelings. This triggers some of my angers.

3. What else is happening now? Could this be the straw that broke the camels back? Have we repressed many other feelings to get through our day, or week, or the month? Now we cannot anymore.

4. Risk. What is on the line? What do I risk if I don't get what I want or feel I need? Can I survive this situation? Will it cost me my job, my marriage, my self esteem?

All of the above come together to cause this conflict. It is not just what the other person did so I now feel angry. Understanding the underlining ingredients to our anger gives us more ability to express our anger with dignity. The better we communicate and the better we know how to actively listen the better the chances this conflict will become an opportunity conflict. One that leaves each of us with our dignity, self esteem, our values, and the knowing the other person while angry still cares about themselves, the solution to this situation, and us.

Anger is like a dance. It can be a waltz, a two step or the jitter bug. Each requires us to apply the skills we are learning to break the cycle of dysfunction. Handling our anger in such a way that we fight with dignity.

It is important for us to consider that all of the above invalidates itself if we are in a dangerous conflict. What constitutes a dangerous conflict? My definition of a dangerous conflict is summed up in the following two examples:

1. The problem is theirs. We have learned how to exercise our ability to separate baggage appropriately. With all maturity we know the problem is theirs. examples are alcoholism, drug addicts, and physically violent people.

What is the most effective way to protect ourselves in these types of situations? I believe it is to listen but not to the point of endangering our life or limb and by finding a way to leave the situation as soon as possible.

2. The problem is us. I want to blame someone else for my feelings, actions, or reactions. I now am putting someone else in the same position I was in in example one.

In either case the conflict has become dangerous because one or both parties is not able to fight with dignity. Fighting with dignity means that I am willing to lay my cards on the table in an open, honest, direct approach in the hopes that the other party is willing to do the same. Resolutions come about through negotiation. This is not the case in a dangerous conflict. No dignity here.

I believe that the most important ingredient in deciding whether or not to pursue trying to negotiate through a conflict would be if the conflict belongs to only one of you you are in a dangerous conflict. If it is their conflict due to any type of holism they are not going to communicate properly. They are not going to listen empathically. Your words will be used against you due to their dysfunction.

IN REVIEW

1. What is the meaning of outerdirected?
2. How do we find out how to use our anger to grow?
3. What common factors are there between this situation and situations in our past?
4. What do we feel immediately before we are aware of our anger?
5. What are we afraid of?
6. Is conflict always negative?
7. Name two basic styles of conflict.
8. How can we tell the difference in types of conflict?
9. How can I use conflict to grow?

To be able to fight with dignity we need to acknowledge the differences between how we handle our anger. Three ways to handle anger are;

1. vent
2. repress
3. process

I learned to tell myself;

I need not vent,
I need not repress
I can process this mess. from Thirteen Blessings of the Twelve Steps.

When we are being aggressive we feel no dignity. We leave others no dignity. When we repress we are being passive. We are left with no dignity. When we are in the processing mode we will do the following things to sort our feelings thus allowing us to fight with dignity if there still needs to be a fight.

1. talk --- talk to someone we trust. Talk into a tape recorder. Talk into a mirror. But talking it out gets it out. Out of our body, into the fresh air of day. We think more clearly. We make better decisions.

2. Write and sort--- this is one of my favorites. We can figure out what the bottom line is about our anger. Then we can approach the other person with a clear cut approach to exactly what the problem is. We can also refer back to our notes at a later time as a reference not as to what they did but as to how we sorted our feelings, how we grew through them, how our child pulled to her heart the precious knowledge of step one. "Here is where I am. This is what I am powerless over. This is where I need to change. God help me in my endeavors to see the real me with clear eyes of understanding. Please remove my shortcomings. Help me to understand why some of my shortcomings remain and what you are teaching me by allowing them to guide me once more through my twelve steps. Where I can practice forgiveness and when to walk away with dignity and when to fight with dignity. Mostly Lord teach me to know the difference. THANK YOU, for how you have led me thus far. "Thou maketh me to lay down in green pastures." and peace and serenity that accompany me due to your guidance. Forever I am thankful that you lead me. "

3. Think

4. Seek information on the subject of our concern. This helps us to understand more realistically with what we are dealing. It helps us to understand the other person's point of view. Understanding is the key to dissipating enough anger that we can handle the rest of our anger in a dignified way. We need not agree but we can speak to each other with respect even when angry.

5. Look for what it is in me that this thing pushes old buttons. By understanding myself I am not going to blame others for making me angry. I will understand why I am

angry, why I feel out of control, why this thing they did bothers me. I am now better able to resolve the current problem with the current person.

In my days of dysfunction I had chosen to repress my anger. I did not want to vent my feelings on others and be responsible for hurting them. I therefore talked myself out of anger. Now, I am happy to say, I talk my way through my anger. The worst thing about attempting to talk myself out of anger is there are no resolutions to our anger. We did not acknowledge them. Others did not acknowledge them. No resolutions are made. This same thing causes the same type of problem over and over again until we are sick of it all.

Processing anger allows me to talk, think, or write, my way through my anger. I know that I benefit from the results. The main result is; BEING FUNCTIONAL. Functional means;

1. resolutions come about for me. Even if the other person is not involved at this point, never is involved, or is uncooperative in working for a solution, I have settled my feelings within me. This is not the same as telling myself, "Don't be angry. They didn't mean it. You shouldn't be angry. Reasonable people wouldn't be upset about such a small thing as this."

Guess what! Reasonable people do get upset by such a small thing as this. Reasonable people, however, do one of two things. They either work through it in their own head or they approach the other party involved and say, "Can we talk. I have been upset by something that happened. I'm hoping we can discuss this together."

2. I come to peace of mind.

3. I come to have a new knowledge of myself. I grow. I now function in the world. Dysfunction is called just what it is because we cannot function in a reasonable way, dealing with the things around us without either minimizing the problem or exploding over the problem. My new knowledge causes me to grow and function.

4. I have come to a new knowledge of a new subject area or a better knowledge of an old subject area. I am becoming a more informed person. This can come from information I took the time to be willing to talk to someone who does have knowledge I need or it may come from personal research I have done. It may come from talking with the person with whom I was upset.

5. I gain ability to approach another person with my anger and handle it constructively.

6. I may gain a friend. I will gain a friend. If I do not gain their friendship I am gaining my friendship.

7. They may not end up a friend but I could earn their increased respect.

8. I earn my respect. I learn that I can handle difficult situations and people with dignity. I improve my ability to carry out these same skills in the next difficult situation.

Keep in mind anger need not be aggressive. Assertive is to share my feelings with others. Aggressive is to vent my feelings on others.

REVIEW

1. What are three different ways to handle anger?
2. What does each method do to you and for you?
3. Which do you feel is most appropriate?
4. What is the difference between talking myself out of anger and talking your way through your anger?
5. In the process of working through anger what are some things each of us can do to come to understand the bottom line premise of why we are angry?
6. What are some benefits of processing our anger?
7. What is the difference between assertive and aggressive?

8. When there is a need to confront the person I am upset with what is meant by fighting with dignity?

AN EFFECTIVE TOOL FOR PROCESSING ANGER

This method of processing anger came to me as I told a friend to draw a line down the middle of a paper and write THEY DID in one column and I FELT in the other. Soon after I would begin to teach a class called Handling Anger Appropriately and my chart would expand. Through the teaching of many classes and examples of everyday situations brought up by my students I came to understand the effectiveness of this type of charting of our feelings.

They Did I felt I Did I can change that too......

I do this exercise in writing. I think ahead about situations that commonly come up. Ones where I allow myself to get angry. I do not do this to control the other person. I do not plan the outcome or force solutions as called by Alanon. This is not so I will get my way. I believe they do what they do, now I feel as I feel, then in times past I react to what they did, thus being controlled by what they did. What I was not doing was stopping to think. Stopping to decide what I would prefer to do. I jump in with a reaction to their reaction. No one is acting as their true self would prefer to act. This is our controlling child, or dysfunctional self reacting or using what is called survivor behaviors to keep from being hurt. We are learning to break the dysfunction of the controlling child. We can now take this situation one step further in our head. We can stop and think how we can change our reaction into an action with which we are comfortable. How would we prefer to act in this circumstance? Although we are changing this I call this the real self. This is how the real self would prefer to act. This is not for the purpose of controlling another. It is for the purpose of fighting with dignity if there needs to be a fight. It is for the purpose of preventing a fight wherever possible without forsaking our rights, boundaries. We are taking our sail out of their wind.

I do this so I can decide a more appropriate action to take the next time a similar situation occurs. In the heat of the moment I cannot think clear. I cannot think of an option that is best for me and others. When I plan ahead I am more likely to put more constructive ways to behave into practice. This is about learning to use the information I have learned. This is called wisdom. Wisdom is the ability to use the information we know in situations that arise in our life.

Use our wisdom in any relationship. Those with our teenagers will be about power. Who decides curfew? Who decides on the final choice of friends?

In the marriage relationship the most common problems are often about power. Who handles the money? Who decides on what car to buy? Who decides if mom works or not? Who decides on child discipline? All are serious questions. We are striving to work out solutions in a functional way. Our resolution process involves several steps. They are;

1. Awareness- We have learned it is okay to be aware of how we feel even when those feelings are negative. The feeling may not be okay. It is however, okay to know we feel it. Now we are in the position to do something about it. Now we can face our true self. Be a spiritual person. Matt: 5:3 "Blessed are they that know their spiritual poverty," Modern Language Bible Yes, we are blessed. Blessed with the knowledge required to grow.

We are now aware we are angry, irritated, or exasperated. These feelings can turn into battles. The conflict is brewing. The sooner we are aware the better the chance for a simpler solution. This awareness allows us to acknowledge the need to settle this issue before other factors get tied up with it and complicate the issue and the solution. The angrier we allow ourselves to get the more likely we will not sound reasonable when we present our side. We may be giving to them our emotional control. Letting ourselves be controlled.

2. Setting limits. Here we decide what point or points are to be argued. Do not try to settle all your differences in this setting. Stick with one principle. For now, this

time, we are working on this. Leave the other problems for another time. After we have come to some sort of resolution in this case it will be more likely we will be able to reach resolutions in other areas. If each party is able to honestly express their need in this area, feel their need is being considered by the other person, and negotiate a solution that each party involved can live with, we will have earned respect from each other. Making future resolution time easier to approach. We have established a level of trust.

If the other person gets involved with bringing in other issues we can say, "that will have to wait until another time. Let's stick with this point." or "I very strongly feel we need to discuss this at this time." Then return to the point you were making. This is part of what is called verbal judo. If the other person keeps coming back to a point we do not want to discuss we can use what is called, "the broken record technique," we just keep saying, "I really want to stick with this subject today." They will eventually get the point.

In step two, setting limits of this debate each person makes a claim for their position. I can state exactly what bothers me. I can say, "when you leave your coat on the coach I get ticked." I can say, "When you read the paper all evening I feel ignored. I would like to talk with you and feel like you are listening."

In constructive conflict we recognize the other person's point of view. Without our empathic listening this situation could end up a verbal free for all. Each person may be returning to their point. Each has a different point to discuss. Each ignores the other. When we show empathic listening we show we care about how they feel. We can say, "I see why you feel that way." You are not saying, "I agree." You are only saying you acknowledge how they feel. They do not have to feel like we do to be okay, acceptable. Here we have broken the prime premise of dysfunction.

Let's say that our oldest teenager has just gotten her driver's license. She now takes her youngest brother out for ice cream and shopping as a fun thing to do. This day he is expecting to go for ice cream after school. The older sister is called into work. He is disappointed. "You promised." he cries. She can respond by saying, "Oh, shut up, you brat." or she can say, "I understand why you are disappointed. Today my schedule has changed and I can't. But I will take you tomorrow. Is that okay?" This statement acknowledges the other person's side and explains her side at the same time. If this does not work we may reach;

3. The Arguing stage. Here areas of disagreement come to the surface. We establish a goal to understand each other better. This understanding comes from both our verbal and nonverbal communication. 93% of our communication is from nonverbal skills.

In the arguing stage each person has a game plan to present his side. Notice the key word is present. Not convince the other. If the conflict is short we move on to the next step. We do not make personal attacks on the other person. This comes under the fight fair rules which will be discussed shortly. Name calling gets people stuck in their anger.

4. Now it is time to negotiate. We bargain with each other. This is common in business. And while people do this day in and out on the job they forget how to do it once they walk out the office door.

Without negotiation there are no resolutions. Negotiation amounts to compromise. Each party comes out feeling, "This was a fair deal." Their needs were met. Each party is willing to talk about what they feel they must have to be happy in this situation. I call this putting all the cards on the table. Not holding a trump card for control. Only when both parties do so can a true compromise be made. Each party is willing to forfeit some points to get what they want in other points. Each party is willing to let the other have some points their way.

Sometimes we think we have reached a successful negotiation only to find out later we cannot live with certain points. Then conflict will arise again. We negotiate again. Sometimes negotiation is not successful. It can be destructive and disappointing. The solution that came about meets no ones needs. Conflict will rise again.

5. Follow up- Here solutions are put into action. Any emotional problems that caused conflict are resolved. If someone felt they were not being considered in this situation and some of their ideas were used or they now understand why a certain idea they had would not work here the cause of their emotional pain is gone. The

resolution process should have increased closeness between the fighters. We are now able to put the disagreement behind us. This allows the relationship to remain strong or grow strong or stronger.

REVIEW

1. What is conflict?
2. List three factors that cause conflict.
3. List five stages of conflict resolution.
4. What is negotiation?
5. When both sides give in a little to reach a solution, what are they doing?

CONFLICT RESOLUTION REQUIRES GOOD COMMUNICATION SKILLS

To prevent or to solve conflict we must develop good communication skills. Since most people have trouble with communication this thought may scare us. Relax! Good communication is developed by learning only a few good skills. None of which are difficult to learn or hard to use.

When we resolve conflicts in a fair way we will improve the quality of our life with our family and our friends. We are becoming more functional and role modeling function for those who like what you do they too may copy some of your examples of communication. The likelihood is we will have more friends. We may lose some friends, I have, but we will gain new and better, more functional relationships. People will be drawn to us as we endeavor to understand others instead of always striving to have them understand us.

You may want to refer back to the Accurate Communication chapter and review listening skills but for the purpose of this chapter we will summarize briefly.

There are several types of listening. They are; passive, selective, active, and reflective. Body language is also of key importance to how we are understood. In brief, some positive body language signals are summed up in the word SOFTEN.

S-smile
O-open posture
F-forward lean
T-touch, hand shake, shoulder pat.
E-eye contact
N- nodding, nurturing.

Soften is the perfect choice of words to represent body language that is conducive to an approachable person and conversation that will deal with conflicts in as dignified a manner as is possible under this set of circumstances.

Women have each of the above tasks easier. Research has showed that women use the plural pronoun more than men-we, you, us. Women enter a session with a question. Women nod their heads more in agreement than men. Women like to trouble talk. Women have a higher need to talk. Women use conversation to bond. All of the skills we are talking about are skills that build communication and bond people together. Even a short relationship like an encounter with a sales person in a store as we return a damaged item is long remembered for how it is handled. We formed an opinion about the person with whom we dealt. She was nice, or what a witch.

HOW LISTENING IS USED TO REDUCE CONFLICTS

In our discussion of listening skills we did not discuss how the active listener differs from a argumentative listener. This chapter is entitled Fighting With Dignity. Let's compare the strategies of the Active Listener with an Argumentative Listener to see how our listening skills will make or break our ability to fight with dignity.

Active Listener	Argumentative listener
listens to content	judges the content through what he already thinks
does not judge the content but listens for the whole message	filters the same information by what he agrees with, misses the whole message
listens to intent of speaker considers intent as responding to the whole message of speaker	judges intent of speaker makes assumptions about the speaker and the message
Sees intent to manipulate audience but refrains from a positive or negative judgment	Focus on intent to manipulate audience and reacts negatively
assesses nonverbal communication	reacts to nonverbal communication "Did you see the way they looked at me?" "I wonder what they meant by that?" "I know they don't like me." "You never can please them anyway."
monitors his nonverbal communication and filters, blocks, preset ideas.	does not monitor nonverbals
responses to whole message and is careful to control the message he is giving to the other person nonverbally. Aware of his nonverbals	responds with his emotions. Does not control nonverbals

listens without judgment Listens with empathy	Listens to judge and evaluate the speaker. If I don't like what you say I don't like you.
attempts to understand your viewpoint	listens to evaluate how you do things. If I don't like how you do things I don't like you.

BARRIERS TO EFFECTIVE LISTENING

We are all just human. We will not get this perfect. Healing from dysfunction is not about becoming perfect. It is about letting go of our need to be perfect. At times we will react and overact. Our reaction will be due to:

1. misreading nonverbals: a speaker may be frowning because of something they thought of and we think they are frowning at us. Before acting or responding take the whole message into account.

2. hidden agendas: everyone has one. Unspoken issues relate to the conversation. These can lead to conflict when they are not discussed openly or when one of the persons feels so strongly he cannot accept the other person's position.

3. Standards and expectations: if the person speaking does not meet our standards this presents capacity for conflict.

4. prejudging - we go into this conversation already having judged what the other person has said. Now is great potential for conflict.

5. emotions against our intellect: when we listen emotionally we will have verbal conflicts.

LISTENING TECHNIQUES FOR HANDLING CONFLICTS.

Our first step is to defuse any argument. We can use a combination of active and reflective listening skills as follows;

1. talk about the behavior, not the person. Do not make this an argument of personalities. Stick to the issues. I can say to my son, "I want you to be home by midnight." If he argues I do not talk about how many times he broke the rule or call him a stupid kid. I simply say, "Sticking to the point, your father and I want you home by midnight. If you are late you will not be allowed to go to the next activity."

2. acknowledge each person is of value. Conflicts are struggles for power. Through active listening I can turn this from a no win situation to a win win situation. Everyone gets something they want. We show respect for their right or value as a person by remembering they have a right to their opinion.

3. Avoid absolutes; you always, you never, overgeneralizing only creates more trouble. If I am told, "You always," I can respond with, "You said, I always do such and such but I feel...." We need to focus on solving the problem at hand instead of focusing on the negatives.

4. Use I messages or I feel messages. I do not say, "You did," Maybe I feel they did and maybe they did, and maybe they didn't. Even if they did, it will be easier to come to a resolution if I can say, I feel....."when you....I felt...." I DO NOT SAY,'YOU

DO NOT KNOW WHAT YOU ARE TALKING ABOUT." I say, "When you talk about several problems at once I get confused.

In regard to curfew problems, I can say to my son, "When you don't get home on time I feel like you are purposely defying me." He said, "I see why you feel that way but mom it really is not on purpose. Most of the time I just don't watch the time close enough." In return, I said, "I think the remedy for this problem is for you to pay better attention to the time. I want you to make an effort to get here on time." Him, "I know that it is my weakness."

5. Use your mind and control your feelings. We do not have to let everything we feel blurt out. Ask myself; what skills do I have that can help here? What solution will work for all of us? What is the problem and what can we change? Do we need additional information?

6. Pick a neutral territory if possible when you think it possible there may be a conflict. Less likely to argue in public.

7. Quickest way is to refuse to participate. I can say, "Let's talk at a time when we can both be reasonable and calm."

8. Avoid distractions so we can actively listen.

9. Control the situation. They may want to discuss it right now. It does not mean we have to. We can schedule this for tomorrow if we feel they have ganged up on us.

10. Enter each discussion prepared to be logical.

11. Use the past as a reference only if need be. Never use it to cast blame.

12. Strive for a win win solution.

All of the above sets of things to do and to listen for may seem complicated. I don't think so. All amount to show respect by realizing each person has the right to be different. No one can undo the mistakes of the past. Don't punish others with their or our past. Try not to force our opinions on them. With these comes another set of rules. These are essential to fighting fair or fighting with dignity. They are:

1. Be assertive not aggressive. Are we out to destroy?

2. Stay in the present. If the issue is something someone continually does then it will be easier to solve if we say, "This is something I'd hope to settle since it keeps coming up. I really need to talk about it."

3. Don't lecture. This will be difficult but with practice it gets easier to make a statement of several sentences that goes straight to the point. State your point as directly as possible. I can say, "The thing I'm upset about is...." or "The point here is." Several advantages to this method. We talk less. The other person is less frustrated. We feel better. We feel understood. Because they are less frustrated they will pay more attention next time. We begin to feel they are listening. We now have growing respect for each party from each party.

4. Listen to the other person. Show true respect. I may with you disagree but I don't try to make you me.

5. Avoid being judgmental.

6. Put active listening into practice.

7. Fight only about one thing.

8. Don't impugn bad motive. Assume the other person wants us to be happy. I think that it is rare that others maliciously hurt other people. Their conduct may be upsetting to us but that does not mean that they planned to do things that hurt us.

9. Take time out if it starts getting heated. This is very important. As we attempt to talk through our problem we will at times get heated. Take a break. Calm down, come back to it. Each time we will work through part of the problem. Relationships improve. If we drop it it is more likely that the problem will arise and arise with more intensity because no resolutions, no compromises were agreed upon. We now have the same fight over and over again.

We are attempting to fight with dignity. All of the above skills will be enhanced as we learn some words to avoid. Eliminating these words is easily done by replacing them with more appropriate wording.

Conflict word	Replacement Word
you	I
but	and
always	this happens at times
can't	will you try
never	I think I don't see this as much as I would like
woulda	I would like to see you do this instead
coulda, shoulda, oughta	I think a good idea is

Let's see the effect of each of the above. Ex. I say to you, "You are my best friend but you should know by now." What is your response? How about, "You are my best friend and I think I'd like to tell you how I feel about...."

"Can't you ever get your work done by deadline?" becomes, "Will you try to meet the deadline?"

"I never see your work turned in on time." to ""I think I don't see your work turned in on time as much as I would like to be comfortable."

"You're always late." "Your being late happens at times. I need you to work for improvement in this area."

I'm sure the few examples listed above give ample enough idea how to set this process in motion. Make a list of things you can rephrase. Things that will help to reduce tension and conflict and still allow you to take care of your needs. Never resort to the silent treatment. No resolution comes from the silent treatment. It is a nonverbal method of saying, "You don't count here." We are working on addressing the issue.

People are most easily irritated when hungry or tired. Alanon uses the statement, HALT, to describe when we need to stop and take care of our feelings. HALT stands for, hungry, angry, lonely, and tired. We can recognize these in ourself and in others. Show respect for them and us. When we show respect in any relationship we try to keep our cool. We have all heard count to ten. While counting I may decide not to be angry. Here are some questions I can ask of myself;

1. Is this so important that I want to risk this relationship?
2. Will this problem be just as big tomorrow? Does it only seem big because I allowed myself to get angry?
3. Am I sure of the facts in this situation? Maybe I can ask more questions, get more information, then decide whether or not to stay mad.
4. Am I acting in a mature way?
5. Am I likely to say something I will regret?
6. Have I made an honest attempt to find a peaceful solution?
7. Will this episode help the situation on the whole or is this only a outlet for my tension?
8. Is there anything humorous in the situation? Can I laugh and relieve some of the tension?
9. Is quarreling becoming a bad habit in this relationship?
10. Could there be a better way to settle my differences?

In considering all of the information on how to fight with dignity I must consider if I create barriers to resolutions. I must also consider how if at all the other person may create barriers to resolutions. Some of which are hitting, pushing, scratching, or any physical action including pulling or throwing by the hair. In addition to physical actions would be a struggle for superiority, a need to be the winner. A spirit of competition which prevails. Is it really possible to work and effective compromise in the grips of a competitive spirit. And I believe perhaps the biggest barrier of all that of control. One that tries to direct the behavior of the other person. One that tries to get this through their thick head, if it's the last thing I ever do. Control, codependence, dysfunction was our barrier to resolution time. Information available today is for the purpose of helping all of us to release degrees of our dysfunction, thus becoming more a more functional. For some of us the ensuing struggle against dysfunction will be harder than for others. Some are afraid of change while others feel liberated by change. We will change as we are ready. Each change we make will help our life to run smoother. Each change we make will bring us to the realization how much dysfunction hurt. How much work we put into changing into mature, functional adult adults will be the best thing that has happened in our life. When we were children we acted as adults to survive. "How mature they are. Way beyond their years," is what we were always told. We were child adults. We grew into an adult. A physical adult, one with many emotions of a child. We were now the adult child. We are now adults attempting to be adults. An adult adult. This is the true mark of breaking the cycle of dysfunction.

In summary of our discussion I would like to say that we, adult adults, are handling our anger effectively, we are sorting our feelings and deciding when not to fight and when we must confront (or discuss) our needs, even if this results in a confrontation we are equipped to fight with dignity. In our process of fighting with dignity we can defuse the conflict by;

1. Not letting others irritate you. Sometime they are deliberately trying to provoke you. You can take your sail out of their wind.

2. Focus on the positive. This may truly not bother you when you look for the positive.

3. Change the subject to something constructive. Lighten up the situation.

4. Take a personal stand against serious conflict, especially physical. Realize this harms people. Work for nonviolent resolutions.

5. Don't let people intimidate you or bully you into fighting. You can show your

strength by doing what you want to do, not what others want or try to control you into doing.

6. Simply walk away. We can say, "Let's talk later when we are calm."

REVIEW

1. How can learning to handle disagreements strengthen relationships?
2. What types of factors cause conflict?
3. What are the stages of conflict?
4. What skills can you use to resolve conflict?
5. How many issues should be addressed at one time?
6. What is respect?
7. Can conflict be prevented?
8. How can we reduce conflict?
9. What is compromise?
10. Why is listening so important to conflict resolution?
11. What is more important a person's words or his body language?
12. What types of things cause barriers to conflict resolution?
13. What might happen if a person represses his anger for too long a period of time?
14. Why must some people win the argument?

THINGS NOT TO SAY TO YOUR KIDS, BETTER WAYS TO SAY WHAT YOU NEED TO SAY

The dysfunctional family does not model a realistic example of how to interrelate within the world. In healthy, functional families, parents encourage sharing of thoughts and feelings and respond to the expressions of each individual. Family members feel free to talk about what's going on with them.

In the dysfunctional family feelings are too painful to acknowledge. Silence and put downs keep everyone from knowing what is going on with another indivuals or the family unit as a whole. This is in essence being told what to feel, what we saw and what we heard were wrong. If you heard fighting in the night accompanied by dish breaking and got up to a clean house with no evidence of a fight we begin to question what we heard.

Healthy families have a regularity to routines and family rituals. These offer consistency and predictability for children with out being so inflexible that our family ritual becomes oppressive.

In the dysfunctional family rules are unclear and often broken. Our very survival depends on our ability to guess what to do next. And hope you guess right. The child's needs are not acknowledged as being different than adult needs.

To teach healthy boundaries we can say to our child; "Yes, that's yours." "Let your sister have her doll back." These types of statements teach a physical boundary as regards material possessions.

Parents still have the most amount of influence on their children. What we want to do is to bring up a moral child. This is done by bringing up a loving child. Parents nurture their children's awareness of others by saying things such as, " Remember that your friend is not allowed to eat sweets, so I don't want you to tease them about having fruit while they are here." We are thus teaching our children to consider the point of view of others. We can do this by asking them on appropriate occasions, "How would you feel if...?" This is not the same as screaming at them, "How would you feel if someone did that to you?" We simply say how would you feel if someone made fun of you for not being able to have ice cream?"

We are now teaching our children to care about how others feel. In our previous chapter we discussed fighting fair. We as parents want to model fighting fair for our children. We have learned it is not how often we conflict that is important but how the conflict is handled that is important. This is a valuable lesson for our children also. The rule in our home is no name calling. Under no circumstances is name calling allowed.

As we the parents are exercising what we have learned about allowing others to express their feelings it is important (vital) that we do not swing too far in the other direction, allowing children to run the house. Children too must learn the art of being allowed to express their feelings knowing they will be listened to and expecting to get everything because they were allowed to express their thoughts and feelings. Again I must go back to my original statement from Profile of Abuse, "I can say, I want, I need or I feel, because I am free to say, I want, I need, or I feel, does not mean I expect to get everything I want, I need or I feel."

As parents we want to allow our children to express their thoughts and feelings then we, as parents, must balance the act by saying, "I 'm glad you told me how you feel but mom and I think...." this can be easily illustrated by the matter of curfew's. Our teenager expressed the thought that since he was 16, had his own car, and earned his own money that we had no say in what time he came home. He felt he had proven his dependability and was capable of deciding for himself when to come home. We stated to him that he was to be home at 11 p.m. Again his presentation of why he could come home at about 2 a.m. if that is what he wished. In keeping with the title of this chapter things not to say to our kids, we did not say, "Listen here young man what gave you the right to decide different than what you are being told. It's 11 p.m. or nothing. Did you hear me?" I did say to him, "Your father and I want you home by 11. We realize you are dependable or we would not let you go at all. You can choose to stay home or be home by 11." "Awe, Mom." was his reply. To which I responded, "If you decide to go and do not get home by 11 the next time you will not be allowed to go." This I said and left the room. This I have learned to do so I do not get caught up in repeating myself and aggravating the situation.

Another example I can think of is when one of our daughters was 16. A friend called her and asked if she could go to the movies. We said she could go but we would have to know what the movie was. We were then told the tiles of two or three movies the girls were considering. All were rated R. Our rule is and always has been, no R rated movies. So we said to her, "If you can pick a movie that is not rated R we will let you go." She said, "I can't tell my friend I'm not allowed to see R rated movies." I responded, "If that embarrasses you don't tell her just say, 'how about.........(name of movie not rated R)?' She decided to tell her friend that she changed her mind and was not interested in a movie that night. All evening she sulked around the house. Finally she said, "I could have gone to the movie with my friend instead of being bored around here." In keeping with what not to say to our kids, we did not say, "We told you you could go. Who's fault is it that you are bored. You have to live by our rules while you are in this house." We simply said, "You're right you could have gone to the movie. It's too bad you decided to stay home."

Along with the above children learn by example that family rules include showing respect for others peoples property, treating others with courtesy, being considerate of parents and elderly persons, telling the truth, keeping your word, not making bigoted remarks or sexist remarks, and not gossiping. These too are set by our example. One of my sons has been a computer whiz since very young. When he was about 12 we got him his own computer. His was the only computer in the house at that time. One day my nephew was here when my son was not home. My nephew asked if he could play a game on Matt's computer. "No, Matt is not here. It is his computer. He is the one that has to give permission to use the computer not I." After Matt got home I told him the above. He said, "Mom it's okay if you let him play on it." "Well Matthew, I don't give anyone permission to use other peoples stuff. So he'll just have to wait to use your computer when you are home." These are ways we demonstrate respect for the property of others.

Other politenesses and boundaries are learned more from example than from word. Unspoken family rules may be;

1. shut the door when you are in the bathroom.
2. knock on the bathroom door if it is shut.
3. respect the answer given when knocking on any shut door.
4. how much clothing is acceptable to walk around the house.
5. when and how we touch each other in the family.

Learning how to break the cycle of dysfunction is about passing on to our children a preferable pedagogy. The Preferable pedagogy is established and passed on to our children by having parenting goals. Here is my list of goals I wanted for my children;

1. To have a good home life. One where they feel important. One that lets

them know they make a difference in this world.

2. A home life that allows our child to want to spend time at home. While at the same time acknowledging that as they grow older and relate more to the world around them they will spend less time at home. But the time spent at home will be a refreshing break from the world outside.

3. An education that will provide them with the skills to follow the life career of their choice. I have a son that is a roofer, a daughter that is a legal secretary, a daughter that is an accountant, a son who is an auto mechanic, and a son who is a radio DJ writes poetry, songs and can entertain a crowd without any advance preparation and entertain them all evening if that is what is required.

4. A home that provides for them a basis for their individual spirituality.

5. An understanding of financial matters.

6. A spirit of cooperation and mutual understand of others.

7. Communication where all are comfortable.

8. A peaceful supportive environment.

9. A sense of personal responsibility and accomplishment. This is achieved by allowing the child to contribute to the family from infancy. Letting them know that what they do makes a difference to the welfare of the family. I strongly believe we are better not to say, "I love you," to the child when they have done a job well. Many years ago I made a conscious decision never to mix I love you with a compliment. I simply say, "I like what you did." or "Thank You." "You did great." "You know what I like about how you did this is......" I will say I love you at another time unrelated to what they have done.

10. The ability to care about others.

11. The ability to make decisions for themselves. Interestingly one of my adult sons recently said to me, "You're not my mom anymore." to which I said, "Why do you feel that way." His reply, "because you don't act like a mom anymore." I said to him, "How I see it is; I am not your mommy anymore. Your mom I will be forever. You are 22 years old and I feel I treat you as the young man that you are. One that is capable of making his own decisions. One that can live with whatever comes from the decisions you make. I love you and care for you. But our relationship is going to be different now than when you were a kid. You were a child and I was an adult. Now we

are both adults and I will listen to what you have to say. However, I hope you don't mind if we talk as the two adults that we are. I think this is my way of honoring your ability to think and make decisions. You are very capable and I trust in your capabilities, as a man." He sat straight up in the chair, his large blue eyes became even larger, his head straightened up as his blond hair softly fell across his forehead. All he said was, "Yeah, okay. I didn't know that." But his body language and the broad smile across his face gave evidence of a new confident thought about himself, how his mother views him, and what relationships are about.

12. Respect for themselves and others. Not walking around in their underwear or opening the bathroom door is part of our respect for others.

13. A strong sense of self esteem.

14. The ability to be honest under all circumstances.

15. The ability to think for themselves.

16. To know the difference between right and wrong.

17. Friends who are positive influences.

18. Joy of heart.

19. The ability to say no to negative actions and things that could hurt them, lying, stealing, smoking, cursing, drugs in any form, and alcohol.

20. Belief in their own abilities. I must show them I believe in their abilities before they can believe in their abilities.

21. The ability to not just see the negative. There is good to be had even from negative circumstances. Even if the good is learning they we can deal with the negative, use the things we learn to create positive circumstances, and use the pain we have felt to be empathic and caring of ourselves and others.

22. The ability to love other people.

23. Good functional relationships of their own. A loving family of their own.

24. Skills to hold a job. Skills to be able to care for themselves in a physical and spiritual way.

25. The ability to set goals. Realistic goals. Not goals that we burden them down.

When we practice Preferable Pedagogy skills we will be giving to our children the above. If we are dysfunctional we will produce dysfunctional children. Even when they do not like our example. They may attempt to be totally different than us. They then are identifying themselves by what they are not instead of what they are. If we teach our children by the good example of functionality we give to them the opportunity to be functional. They may not be functional. They may decide to act differently than what was modeled for them. They do however have the choice between being functional or dysfunctional. They do know functional when they see it. They can emulate the above qualities if they choose. All of the above reflect good levels of self esteem.

The things we say and do not say to our children make or break their ability to view themselves through the confident eyes of a growing person with abilities and skills, thoughts and feelings, ones that are theirs, even if they are different than the thoughts and feelings of those they love.

What we say and don't say makes the difference in their thought process and their level of self esteem. Here I would like to list what I believe to be the most common statements expressed by adults to children. Ones that erode away self esteem or prevent the building of self esteem.

You never listen.
Can't you do anything right?
How many times have I told you?
Close the door. Were you born in a barn?
You're the clumsiest thing I've ever seen.
You're just like your father (or anyone else with a negative connotation.)
When will you ever learn?

Are you stupid?
Children should be seen and not heard.
Can't you be more responsible?
I expected better of you than that.
You're lazy.

You're impossible!

You're just not cut out for that.

You couldn't do what I have to do. I've done it every day for years. You couldn't hold up under what I have to put up with.

You can try it but I don't thing it's going to work.

You'll be the death of me yet!

I don't know why I put up with you.

You were an accident anyway.

Just this once, try to tell the truth.

You're always in a bad mood.

I can't stand your laughing. That wasn't funny. You are crazy.

You always interrupt.

You always talk when you should be listening.

Haven't I taught you anything?

I'll get this through your thick head if it's the last thing I ever do.

I'm at my wits end with you.

Why should I listen to you?

Why should I believe you?

Why should I trust you?

Why should I give you another chance?

You're just no good at that! Give up!

Your brother or sister never talks like that!

Do you understand what I have to do everyday because of you?

I don't want to hear another word out of you.

All you ever do is complain. I've got my own problems.

This time try to get it right for a change!

Who do you think you are?

Your room is always a mess!

You have no respect for anything.

You're always getting into something.

You just don't think, never have.

This is the last time I'm going to tell you.

I can talk to you until I'm blue in the face and it doesn't do any good!

Where were you when the brains were being passed out?

Nothing I say makes any difference to you. It just goes in one ear and out the other!

Do any of the above sound familiar? I think we have all heard them all. All of these are things not to say to our children and while we are at it we can stop saying them to ourselves. We are learning to break the cycle of dysfunction. We are giving ourself credit for the good things we do. We are saying, "Job well done." "I like the way I..." We are erasing old parental tapes. The tapes that depowered us. The tapes that were taught by means of the poisonous pedagogy down through millenniums of time.

All of the above quotes I refer to as verbal abuse. We can be abused without any of the above verbal appendages being directed our way. Abuse ranges from emotional, verbal, physical, and sexual with varying degrees in each category. Without verbal abuse being present we may be emotionally abused. Emotional abuse does not contain any of the above statements. It is not an overt act of mistreatment. While I attended Codependents Anonymous I saw that those who were not verbally, physically or sexually abused had trouble putting their figure on what the problem was. To this we can come to understand the eroding away of the soul that occurs with emotional abuse.

It is not only what is said to each of us that gives messages to our subconscious. What is not said is just as powerful as what is said. Our need as a child is to know we have skills and abilities that make a difference that we are here. We are important. The most important feeling we will ever have. Emotional abuse occurs when this need is not fulfilled. The lack of filling our child soul results in an emotionally wounded soul who's body grows to be an adult while the soul is still that of a hurting child. The hurting child is longing to hear the following;

That was really great!

I'm proud!

You did it!

You were wonderful!

You really do that well.

You worked so hard.

As always, you look good today.

You're a winner!

I trust you.

I can always count on you.

You're really smart.

People really like you.

I like the way you did that.

You're really fun to be with.

I feel good when I'm with you.

You really take responsibility for yourself.

I appreciate your honesty.

I like the way you keep your room neat.

You've improved in how you make your bed.

You have lots of energy.

You're really positive.

I feel good seeing you laugh.

You always seem to keep yourself busy.

I like your creativeness.

You got the best of dad and me.

I'm so happy I can rely on you.

That was close. Next time will give you another opportunity to try again.

Good job!

You're beautiful.

I like the way you put that outfit together.

You're really very pretty.

You're handsome.

You're my favorite three year old boy in the world.

I love your smile.

I listen to what you say.

I like you as a friend.

I like the way you get along with the other kids.

You're an achiever.

I 've noticed how well you listen.

It's obvious that you care about people.

I glad you took time for yourself.

You made track. Hey!

I'm proud of how you do in school.

You're special to me.

Much better. You can do it!

You made that look so easy. I have a hard time with it.

I love you and I like you.

I appreciate your good manners.

There is no one like you in all the world.

You sure are talented.

Good answer.

Thank you.

I sure appreciate your thoughtfulness.

You deserve it.

Can I help?

The absence of these and other positive statements are covert acts that leave a child feeling no one cares if he or she is here or not. Do we make a difference? Does it matter that I am here? What would happen if I died? Would they miss me? All questions that plague the hurting child.

There are other things we say to ourselves and our children that are covert acts of emotional abuse, dysfunction. We communicate to our children by what we do and what we do not do. We create negative feelings within our child if we;

1. Always look too busy to be approached.
2. Do not show up for an important event.
3. Use physical force.

4. Lose control or throw things.
5. Frown when they speak to us.
6. Leave the table because of an argument.
7. Storm out of a room.
8. Drive recklessly because of anger.
9. Make promises and then break them.
10. Put things off.
11. Don't take the time to talk to them one on one.
12. Do not take time out for family time.
13. Lye or ask children to lye.
14. We do things we do not want our children to do.

Children learn from our example. We are not perfect. We are endeavoring to do the best we can. We may not always be able to avoid frowning when someone else speaks to us. We can make it a practice not to lye. Think of the impact of a parent punishing a child for lying and then asking a child to say they are younger than they are to get a movie ticket cheaper. These things are inexcusable bad modeling.

All of the negative talk we are eliminating as we speak to the next generation is best modeled if we practice all of the same standards as we talk to our inner child. Our hurting child of long ago. It was and is our hurting child that has brought us to the road of recovery. We seek to break the cycle of dysfunction as we want to give to our offspring the benefits of a preferable pedagogy. Give it to ourselves. Show them the value of loving ourselves. Not loving ourselves more than others as is promoted in me-ism. Model to them the love of self that Jesus, himself spoke about when he said, "Love your neighbor as yourself." This love encompasses loving ourself in a way that we know we are important, other people are important, we are not more important than others, we are not less important than others. This is functional. This is the ability to express our needs, acknowledge our feelings, model to our children it is okay if they too express their needs, acknowledge their feelings, care for others without caretaking others, know they are important, know the joy of knowing they do make a difference in this vast universe.

Every time I treat myself well, every time I forgive myself, every time I treat my child with respect, and honor him/her as a human being I am breaking the cycle of dysfunction. I am expressing my cycle of function, my preferable pedagogy by noticing what is right. I must take time to notice things my children do that is right. I must look for positive actions on the part of my child. Then I comment about what I see. Keep track. Look for ten things your child does each day that you like. Write them down. Ex. He smiled at me when I came in the room. He fixed a chef salad for supper. He apologized for how he talked to me. He asked for a ride to the barbers but asked me if that would make me late. Children crave praise. We became dysfunctional because we didn't receive emotional strokes in our childhood. We thus felt empty. We were still looking for acceptance. Our part of breaking the cycle of dysfunction for our children means we must verbalize what we see in them that we like. For a compliment to be accepted to need to be specific. We can say, "I like how you watered the plants. Just the right amount of water." "Thanks for doing the dishes." "Thanks for helping me." "I appreciate you picked up your toys." "Good Job! Your room looks great."

Generalizations do not confirm to the child his worth. Every child needs to know it makes a difference they are here. Just as we, adults, gain satisfaction from knowing we have contributed to the well being of another so does a child. The child contributions need to be age appropriate, however, even in infancy our self worth is established by knowing we make a difference. Generalizations do not build self esteem. "Good boy/girl." "You're so helpful." "I love you. You help me so much."

I think it ironic that when we tell someone, any age, they are good they feel it is because of what they do where as we compliment the things they do and they as a person conclude they are good, they are worthwhile, they are needed. To raise self esteem make specific comments about specific things you have noticed.

1. You made your bed without being asked. Thank You.
2. You cleaned up your own mess, I'm proud.
3. You picked up your toys, thank you.
4. You got an A on your history test, I knew you could do it.
5. A, "one," in conduct. Good job.
6. You tied your own shoes. Great!

7. Your shoes are on the right feet. You're getting good at it.
8. Boy, I feel good. You smiled at me when I came in.

Add to this list anything you notice your child did. It need not be as good as you would like. Give them credit for the effort. Give them credit for any improvement. "You made your bed better than before. Keep it up." To be even more effective add your child's name to the statement. "Matt, you made supper. I really appreciate it." "Matt supper looks great. Thank you." "Matt, I caught your school radio station. You really are a good DJ." Here I would like to contrast some statements of emotional verbal abuse and functional.

No one who is capable needs training wheels.
Hey! You rode ten feet without training wheels. Better. Much better.

Your fund raiser isn't going good.
You sure got grit. You really hang in there even when it's not going so good.

When I was 7 I was the star of the class.
You are doing good. Your reading is improving.

In addition to direct compliments we can build self esteem in our children by;

1. Passing on to them positive comments others make about them. Aunt Jane noticed how well you looked after little Susan. Miss Smith told me your hand writing has greatly improved. The principle called to tell me you are getting a good citizenship award.

2. Let your child hear you tell another parent or teacher something positive about them. Tell one of their friends something positive about them where they can hear.

3. Act in a way to demonstrate love and respect. When driving turn off the radio when they speak. When Matt, my youngest, was about 7, I had a delightful surprise one day as I took him to school. He started to speak, I turned off the radio and he looked at me very pleased. He said, "Do you know what I like about you?" Full of surprise I said, "No, what?" "You turn off the radio whenever I start to talk." he said. "That's because you are important to me." "I know," he said with a big smile.

Sit or Kneel to be able to make eye contact with your child. When going out to a movie or to eat out, ask them their preferences. If you decide to go elsewhere let them know you appreciate their suggestion.

4. Compliment each child once a day for the first week. Don't overdo it. Too much feels phony. The second week compliment them twice a day for the week. The third week 3-4 times a day. This will set a pattern of looking for the positive.

Showing our interest in our child does not mean sharing all our life with them. It also means listening to their life. Open the conversation with a question to show interest in them and their life. If you ask, "What's up?" the answer will probably be, "nothing." We and they will share more fully when we ask open ended questions. Questions that begin with, how, what, when, where, and why. We can also say, tell me about........ Do not settle for one word answers. Illustration;

What's your science project going to be?
"Bones."
"What specific aspect of bones is of the most interest to you?'

Why do you want to go camping?

What happened when you presented your history report?

What was the best thing that happened today?

Too open ended of a question leaves a void. "Tell me about your trip." is asking for too much information to sort at a moments notice.

Ask instead, "What was the best part of your trip?" "Where did you go on your trip?" "What places did you see that you'd like to tell me about?"

One of the largest parts of our dysfunction was the mislabeling of feelings. In passing on to the next generation accurate labeling, accurate feelings, knowing it's okay to feel whatever we feel, we can label for them in our conversation what we see.

child; Johnny hit me!
parent; I see, you're mad at Johnny.
child; I just wanted to play with his truck. He wouldn't let me. I hate him.
parent; So you feel he doesn't like you because he didn't share with you.
child. Yeah!
parent; So you're angry.
child; No! I'm sad.
parent; That face looks angry to me.

In addition to labeling a feeling we teach empathy and caring for others in simply conversations with our child and/or teenager.

child; I'm really nervous about driver's Ed.
parent; Something new can be scary.
child: I've never driven before so I am scared.
parent; I was scared the first time I drove a car.
child; You were.
parent; I think everyone is.
child; Thanks for telling me. I feel better.

We are giving to our teenager the right to be nervous. The function to feel whatever they need to feel. The function of being able to admit to others as well as themselves they are afraid. The validation of knowing they are not not good enough because they are nervous. We are giving them our time, attention, validation, skills, confidence, and the joy of knowing they have limits without feelings that their limits label them as defective in some manner. We are passing on to them the joy of breaking the cycle of dysfunction.

SETBACKS

I was almost finished writing Profile of Abuse when I experienced what will probably be one of many setbacks. At that time I added to my chapter on anger a section I called The Cycle of Repressed Anger. I wrote that section based on nothing but my own feelings.

Our setbacks come upon us sometimes because we're trying too hard. I had become in the process of learning how to not control self conscious about everything I considered saying. All my life I felt I had walked on eggs. In my mind I would now say, "Is this control? Now I was getting angry. Why? I felt controlled. Do not say, do not do, anything to hurt anyone. I need to be me! How can I relax, be me, and make sure I don't control. How could I get balanced. It takes time, we will have setbacks . When we do we can remind ourselves about the myths we once believed about anger and why we repressed. Discussed in our chapter ANGER PAST AND PRESENT. These principles can be applied to any and all of our old ways of thinking, feeling and behaving that come from our old dysfunction.

I think that we finish our business, understand why we felt and feel the way we did and do, and learn appropriate ways to deal with our feelings, then for the rest of our life we strive to apply what we've learned. We strive for balance, but balance is perfect, I'm not. We will have setbacks.

As we are learning to be more functional we are met with anger from others who are not ready for and do not understand change. "Anyone from a dysfunctional family that is trying to be their own self will be met with anger and rejection. They must be made to feel guilt. In their family individuals exist for the sake of the family. The family is not there to meet the emotional needs of the individual." Profile of Abuse.

We've detached. They haven't. In our human imperfection we cannot detach 100% 100% of the time. We let things others say and do influence us and even control us at times. But we can learn from it. Write out a list of changes we need to make and how we can go about that, just like we did in our original recovery work. Work through our twelve steps, read self help books. Do research. Use a setback to learn what we may have missed.

Have we rescued? Are we well down the road of recovery? Do we now relapse more by feeling guilty that we are not doing recovery? Have we allowed ourselves to get caught up in Karpman's Drama Triangle? In my times of setback I can;

1. Realize I know what the problem is. I know I allowed others to use me.
2. Know it was my inability to say no that caused my problem.
3. When I then resent and act crazy, yelling and making a scene, I know I am not back to square one. I am back to step one.

In square one;

1. I did not know why I felt crazy and resentful when I tried to help others.
2. In square one I did not know how to separate baggage.
3. I felt unloved and used.
4. I did not know how to say no.
5. I felt guilt for my feelings and my actions.

I am back to step one. I need to come to recognize what I have no power over and what I can change. I setback. I reacted. I didn't say No. I failed to enforce a boundary. I am not perfect. We as imperfect people will not do recovery perfectly. We will have slip ups.

SLIP UPS

I work to be no more codependent.
I slip a little, "I'm codependent for sure."
Sometimes, I feel cured.
Other times, not again my ugly friend.
I thought of you as gone,
Don't show your ugly head.

Every time you come around.
I talk to you and say,
"I told you, I'll not control again like yesterday."

"I know," you say, "but I just thought."
Controlling self, please go away,
I'll not return to yesterday.

from POEMS AND GROWTH FROM ME TO ME

Setbacks may last two minutes. They may last months. We may be reacting to other peoples dysfunction. We may be reacting to ourselves, our previous setback has created a downward spiral within us. We may be reacting to our old dysfunction and years of old dysfunctional habits.

Sliding back into old habitual ineffective habits is a setback. If we have been neglecting ourselves, taking care of others, we will feel victimized. We have had to repress our feelings, numb them, to continue with life. When we cannot anymore we will overreact, try to control, feel dependent and needy, feel guilt for our feelings. We feel afraid. Afraid of further relapse. Afraid all of our recovery work has been in vain.

We feel obligated to others, depressed, certainly deprived, unworthy and trapped.

Setbacks are a normal part of life. Consider the case of a marathon runner who has trained for years, gets into the race, and falls. Our runner does not go back to start. If he falls backward then he gets up and goes on from where he is. At first it will be difficult to continue with perhaps a soar knee, aching hands or whatever was hurt in the fall. Go on they must. Further down the line our runner feels the joy of having continued the race.

This is the process of recovery. We slip. We fall. We are not going backward. We are not back to start. We have failed to uphold our boundaries, our fall. We will get back up and go forward. We know the skills to use. We did it in our original recovery.

I have found myself. I'll stay me. Sometimes in the midst of it all I'll loop around to see what my controlling child can teach me, tire of it all, return to my natural relaxed part of me. Still be me. Relapse, learn, grow. Be me again.

TRIGGERS TO A SETBACK.

Have we let go of control at home and on the job? Are our boundaries well established? We may find that we have well established boundaries in one area of our life and have difficulties in another area.

In recovery for three years I hired into a new job. Soon I began to feel crazy. I felt rejected, unincluded, and negative about my abilities. I began to wonder what was wrong with me. For two months I struggled with why am I feeling this way? The day came when someone in the lunch room asked, "How do you take it working under.....? She's such a party girl, a control freak. How do you keep your sanity?" I replied, "Thank You. I suppose I try to keep my mind on my work." Relief at last. Was I nuts? NO! My codependent negativities flared. Working in an atmosphere of alcoholics or abusive others triggers the same dysfunctional setup that was spurred on in our original dysfunction. Would it be any wonder that being in the same type of situation would trigger the same feelings. I came to apply a principle that continues to help in any dysfunctional situation, regardless of how long I have been in recovery. It is:

In recovery I learned that the responses I had were normal responses to the additive behavior of others. I am as normal now as I was then. If I allow myself to stay in dysfunctional systems my negativities will return. I now need to recognize the problem.

When I start to question, "what is wrong with me?" I need to slow down, take an honest look--yes at myself, and also at the entire situation. What are the realities of this job circumstance, the dysfunction or function level of those with whom I must associate to hold this job.

We learned in our dysfunctional family of origin how to survive it's own set of rules and personality. Employment settings are similar. In an employment setting it may be a single individual who is dysfunctional or it may be the employment system itself.

One of my immediate reactions when I became aware of rampant alcoholism among the supervisors of this particular corporation was to feel I would not be driven out. I could do my work, have my own friends and so be it. Soon I would learn that although my negativities had greatly diminished I would return to my true recovered self when I left that place of employ.

Our setback may be a clue to something we need to work through. It may also be an indicator of how much we have grown. Our growth is indicated as we begin to notice the unhealthy patterns among our co-workers. Yesterday I was told that I was liked better before I got into all this recovery stuff. In the discussion that persuaded the issues discussed amounted to my ability to state what I need from any given situation. This was related to me as selfish. I have grown. Others stayed in their dysfunction. I need not setback. I can remember I have no control over others. They will grow when they are ready. I to stay in their approval would need to setback to their way of thinking. My new level of function requires that I as soon as I am aware of a feeling to connect with my core, my inner child and say, "what do I need here?" I do not need to be a victim because they are a victim.

As I grew this person's anger at me was plain for all to see. Others noticed. Some asked, "What's up with so and so?" My reply, "I suppose you would have to ask her."

Setbacks can occur anywhere people congregate. In religious circles, social circles, professional or charitable associations, and support groups. Wherever people are.

We learned how to take care of ourselves. When we become aware of what feelings of dysfunction are reoccurring we need to deal with those feelings by doing what is required to take care of ourselves. We may;

1. Look for another job.
2. Change religious congregations or support groups.
3. Figure out how to stay functional in the job or congregation where we are.
4. Learn to let go of the pressure of what others think.

I attended Alanon for quite some time. I quit attending and felt very comfortable with my recovery program. Then due to changing circumstances my husband and I decided to reattend. Upon returning the statements made were, "Welcome to our come backers." "You can't do this without our program." and "so you decided to return to recovery."

I thought I appreciated this was only their opinion. But weeks later I was still expressing anger to my husband about the idea that I was not working recovery because I didn't attend group. I needed to let it go. I came to understand that I had outgrown the group. I worked a good recovery program. After getting through my rough spot I again quit attending. Months later several students walked into one of my classrooms, the one called Handling Anger Appropriately. We both laughed. "Well, hello." At the end of the class sessions we walked out together one evening and the man said to me, "What I have to say to you is, you work a very good recovery program. Your class has really helped. I'll take any class you offer." I said, "Thank you."

We can setback in recovery groups if we become dependent on the group. Twelve step groups are a necessary part of recovery. We can however use the groups approval as a substitute for an approving parent. True healing, true functionality requires we establish automomy. We bond and heal as the group serves as a family of understanding, one we never had. Here it becomes important for us to decide,

1. Can we improve in our level of function by staying in this group?
2. Is this group contributing to my dependency needs?
3. Do I need to leave the group to see how I handle myself, my life and my function without the group?

As we had myths about anger as well as all other feelings we will also find we are holding myths about recovery. These myths will reoccur with each setback. Those that are particularly tied to our past style of dysfunction will trigger a setback or reappear with each setback. The more perfectionisticly oriented we were the more these myths appear. Consider the following myths. Each is followed by a suggestion for improvement.

1. I should be doing better than this. Eliminate the word should from our vocabulary. I should have becomes, the next time I will. In times of setback I can say, "Okay I goofed up I think the next time I am in a situation similar to this I will......"

2. I've been working recovery for some time I shouldn't have these problems. Again we find the word should. I can change, "I shouldn't be having these problems," to

I am a normal person.
As normal as ever,
I won't be perfect,
in any endeavor.

3. Working a good program means I wouldn't be doing this. To this I can only say, there is a difference between good and perfect. We cannot work a perfect program. We can work a good program. However to consider one definition of perfect is for this thing to be well suited to the purpose for which it was intended. Using this definition my recovery is perfect. It is perfect for me to learn what lessons my recovery and my God know I need to learn. My lesson will keep appearing until I connect with what it is my God wants me to learn. My program is perfectly suited to me.

When writing Thirteen Blessings of the Twelve Steps I worked for weeks on a chapter only to erase it. I started over. Frustrated with every word. I finished it and thought it distasteful. I continued to work on the book. About a month later in my proofreading of finished copy I came to see chapter eight was very good. Why had I thought it not to be so? It did not live up to what I had in mind at the time. It did not live up to what I thought was a better example. In applying this principle to setbacks I think we may not have setback as badly as we think. We may be comparing this situation to a time when we were working at prime. I cannot always be prime. I always do my best but m y best for today may not be as good as my best of yesterday.

4. If I am a professional in the field I must not have this problem. What if my clients find out? I can delightfully say that as I see the faults of my therapist I can find comfort in knowing they too are people. People who are working their recovery to the best of their ability. I can find comfort in knowing it was a real live person who listened to my pain, who had tears in their eyes, and sometimes a lump in their throat as they too know the pain, hard work, and joy of recovery.

5. I wouldn't be doing this if my recovery was real. I remember well the first time this hit me. I felt like it was like everything else in my life, something which is not what we had hoped it to be. This is a normal response to let down. Every time I know something is normal I can have the satisfaction of knowing to normal problems come normal solutions.

6. People would not respect me if they knew the things I think and feel. Knowing the things another thinks empowers each of us to lend to another the power of recovery. No matter what you think or feel someone has felt it before. Someone will hold you and cry with you. Someone will give to you feedback and respect your ability to decipher what parts of that information you need to continue in your recovery.

7. I thought this one was gone. I did it again. Remember please, old habits die hard and reappear from time to time.

8. I know better than this. We also knew the patterns of dysfunctional thinking and acting for a much longer period of time than we have been working on recovery. I must realize that the real me will mess up. Am I entitled less than any other human that walks this earth?

I am entitled to be me. Let go and let God. We are entitled to make mistakes, to think negative, and thank God we do sometimes. If we could always do right, think right, feel right, how would we know it was right? Matt 5;3 says, "Happy is the man conscious of his spiritual need." Without mistakes would I be aware of my need to look to someone greater than myself, someone to whom I can turn over my cares, someone who can bring sanity into my life?

After we have addressed our personal myths about setbacks and recovery we can now go about reestablishing the rules we set for our own self care. Ask myself "What must I do?" Mine are;

1. I need not be a victim because they are a victim.
2. I have associates that are codependent but I need not bite into their codependency.
3. I will deal with my feelings as soon as I am aware of what I am feeling.
4. When I feel crazy or negative I will stop, take time to think, try to determine what is at the root of my free floating anxiety, anxiety not associated with a certain thing.
5. I will set boundaries and communicate them to the others with whom I associate.
6. I will detach when I feel it necessary to maintain my level of function.
7. I can spend money, time, and care on myself.

I Cor 15: 33 says, "Be not deceived: evil communication corrupt good manners." KJ. Translation.

"Do not be misled. Bad association corrupt good morals." Modern Language.

"Don't be fooled by those who say such things. If you listen to them you will start acting like them." Living Bible

"Do not be deceived: "Bad company ruins good morals." Revised Standard.

I have included four different translations as I found the application to dysfunction quite interesting. The scripture does not say that negative association will effect and affect you if you are not doing your part correctly. It says, you will be affected and effected by negative association. Take a good look at our friends, our associates, our work mates, our job situation. Do your best to associate with healthy people. Other dysfunctional people can set off a trigger (one of our old messages). Take a good look. Remember our primary tool, detachment. Now seek healthy associates, work for healthy behaviors. I find it interesting to note that behavior can be defined as an outward expression of our inner attitude and true personality. Reflected both by conduct and appearance. This is not to say our behavior will be perfect as we would like it. I think the majority of our behavior is what best reflects what we are. Dysfunction is a part of us all. Not a part we are happy about but still a part. A part of us we lived for many years. I think for the rest of my life I will at times setback. I will at times have a visit from my controlling child. I will recognize her, talk to her, listen to her, she taught me many skills. Not all of what she did was wrong. She helped me to survive and to become more and more functional. It was only by becoming functional that I could now survive my survivor behaviors. My controlling child in her control always knew how to survive. In recovery she still knew and loved the real me she had been protecting all those painful years. In recovery she too was willing, sometimes more than others, to show interest in the survival of my true self. She taught my true self how not to give up on recovery. She knew how to get up again when I thought all was for naught. I came to love that frightened little child who learned how to control. She in her control loved the real me enough to protect me. She now knew it was time to say, "goodbye," with just an added thought. "Can I visit now and then?"

She may come to visit when facing conflict, when we are threatened by the thought or suggestion of a loved one leaving, paying bills, hearing a familiar song, hearing someone's voice, anything that reminds us of then and them.

Problems trigger setbacks as they trigger past memories of similar problems and how we were treated in the process of trying to cope with those problems. Success also can cause us to control and caretake. We have learned how to handle problems similar to us but success may be something new. What do I do now, things are changing. Any change of circumstance requires that we take time to take care of ourselves and our needs before setback occurs. Accept our new situation even be it success. Serenity means I accept the things I cannot change. Self compassion is the courage to change the things I can. Take care of myself. Set boundaries. In my new found success I will be in a learning process. What boundaries do I need in this situation? What are my limits? What are my priorities?

The answer to the above questions will get us out of the mire when we feel struck with or in a certain situation or feeling. Sometimes to my shock I am deep into a setback before I recognize it as a setback. "After all this work," I say. Basically meaning, "I shouldn't be doing this. I know better." Go back to my own words, eliminate should from my vocabulary. Remind myself how I can recognize the signs of a setback.

1. Feeling like, I shouldn't be doing this.

2. Have anxiety without knowing why.
3. Talking too much. Not being able to get to my point.
4. Feeling Used.
5. Always being tired. I've overcommitted again.
6. Wanting to run from those abusive in their speak instead of using the new skills I have learned.
7. Feeling guilty about having ambivalent feelings.
8. Being over sensitive.
9. Feeling under appreciated.
10. Sacrificing where sacrifices are not needed.
11. Having difficulty thinking clearly.
12. Not wanting to think for myself.
13. Mind racing.
14. Feeling resentful.
15. Repressing my anger.
16. Abandoning my routine.
17. Doing for others what they can do themselves.
18. Trying to get this chapter perfect.
19. Thinking it's all their fault.
20. Feeling I have no choices.

We will begin to feel better as soon as we identify what we feel and why we feel it. If I feel crazy I can say, "I'm not crazy but something around here is." Look to see where dysfunction is showing.

We may be protecting ourself from new revelations. Even though I have long finished my business I have found in the last six months that almost daily new revelations come to me through new memories. Each time I am shocked at the vast storehouse of memories that come my way. One day while standing at the sink drinking a glass of water, bang a memory, supposedly out of the blue. "Well, I'll be. That's what was going on. That's what this is about. Okay." New insights about life and myself. But my process of recovery has brought me to the point that these months of unfolding truths do not shake my boots. Sometimes I cry. I cry with the understanding of what is happening and how this information relates to circumstances in my life. These tears are happy tears of recovery. I am always thankful for the day I went to therapy and started my process of knowing where and how to find answers. How to go about looking at myself and the events in my life. How to use them for growth and maturity. How to use setbacks to my advantage. I am not trying to recoup my losses. Recovery means I accept my losses and accept the gains that come about through or because of my losses. As I accept this gain is the result of this loss, I gain, get up from the setback I may be feeling due to grief. Grief over my losses is lost. I can now play, laugh, rest, recoup the spirit that recovery has brought to me.

Listen long and hard to ourselves. Our gut knows what the problem is. I can say, "In my gut I feel ....." I have my answer. I can say, "the bottom line here is I feel used when you watch while I work." whatever the case may be. The greatest thing I learned from setbacks is;

WHY I NEED SETBACKS

Writing has always been the best form of releasing pent up feelings for me. I believe it will always be. Writing things out has another advantage over releasing issues of the present and enabling us to sort through our feelings coming to the bottom line. What the problem is at this time. A distinct advantage of writing is that we can draw on the things we have written. During a serious setback I read some of my old notes. I learned what I needed to know now from what I had written many months ago. I had no memory of what I had written. I cannot remember everything I thought or felt.

My issue had to do with forgiveness. I at one time wrote:

I can forgive you without liking you.

If I continue to dislike another person we may believe we haven't forgiven. This is not the same.

It is harder to forgive when the other person has not sorted their baggage. They keep blaming us for their perceptions. That is where detachment comes into the picture.

Every time I am having a setback I realize it is one thing that is the problem. The

problem is: I have failed to detach from their emotions and/or perceptions.

I can forgive you for not forgiving me.

from 1475 CONCLUSIONS OF A HEALING CODEPENDENT.

To honor another means to hold as precious. Be it father, or mother, or anyone else to honor them means to try to understand them, to have empathy for them. It does not mean, I agree. It means I understand. Each setback is my lack of detachment. My lack of detachment is due to confusing empathy with agreement. Each setback is due to my feelings of anger in resistance to a situation or a person whom I feel is attempting to control this situation or myself. Each setback is due to my anger when I feel judged for healing.

I feel I am trying to understand. They push. I feel forced. I do not detach to the extent needed to separate their rights from my rights or I separate my rights from theirs but feel anger when I feel they are attempting to step on or over my rights, boundaries. I regress, setback.

All this I learned not from books, not from counselors. I learned this from setbacks.

I am trying to be as fair as I know how to be. I am trying to forgive. Sometimes forgiveness comes slow and hard. I would venture to say most of the time forgiveness comes slow and hard. Sometimes I do better than others. Sometimes I press ahead with little effort. Sometimes I forge ahead with all the strength I can muster. Other times, I regress.

All this I learned from setbacks.

I can detach in any situation and from any person on this earth with whom I feel my life will improve through detachment. In each case I have decided how I benefit from this detachment. My benefit is not becoming negative, not regressing, not letting setbacks run or ruin my life. I can handle my life in a way to copy the example of a sailor who uses a skill called tacking. Tacking is the ability to weave a ship in and out of the wind. The ability to take our sail out of their wind. Weaving in and out of the wind produces a course that is not straight. A steady charge into the wind with a full sail will tear the sail to shreds. We too can plan our course. Weaving along the way, in and out of the winds of recovery. Our sails will be tested. Our course will be slightly altered. Altered in a way to give us strength to sail back into the winds of recovery accepting each new step as the challenge it was meant to be, one that provides us strength and recovery wisdom.

I need setbacks because I am a normal person, an average person. Average people have ups and downs. All people have ups and downs. Anyone who says they don't is lying, either lying to themselves or to you or both.

I am human. I am real. My setbacks remind me that I have limits. Having limits keeps me healthy in a physical and emotional way. I have not nor will I do anything perfect. This includes recovery. When I remember my limits I am helped to have a more realistic view of myself. I cannot do it right all the time. If everything went right we would never know if we were able to enforce our boundary, improve communication, separate baggage correctly, or grow. If things always went right how would we know if we had grown. Grown in maturity, grown in abilities, grown in forgiveness.

Setbacks enable me to see what it is I need to work on. I can learn how effective my skills are. A setback may also allow me to see how much less severe this setback is compared to the severity of a similar setback of the past. From this we can see how much better we are handling things, even if we are not totally pleased with what we did, we will be able to see our growth if only we give ourselves this opportunity. We can discipline, train, ourselves to work on the areas needing the most attention. My philosophy is; Don't be too hard on yourself. We do not need to tackle everything that we did not do totally right. Analyze the thing we think is the underlining cause of most of our setbacks, work on that quality. As we improve our setbacks will be less and less often as well as less severe.

I would say in times past, "back to square one." Remember how bad square one was. We were in denial. We did not know that our past abuse was the cause of our current problems. We did not know what to do or how to do it. I believe that as long as I do not deny my problems I am not back to square one. I will repeatedly return to step one, realizing where I am powerless, moving through steps two and three bring me to know my God will give me sanity if I let Him.

I do not have to beat myself because the circumstances of this particular time in my life may be harder to deal with than other times of my life. When under stress for any reason we are likely to setback to one degree or another. These are the times when our controlling child will say, "I remember this. I know how to handle this. Let me!" Through recovery I have learned how to be able to say to her, "Thank you, I remember those skills. I can use this point in a different way. I can use the determination and strength you taught me to know I can stick this out. However, I think instead of control I will wait and see if this action is necessary on my part." I can say, "If I'm feeling stupid I know it is a replay of old tapes. I know this is not true. You taught me. At this time I have gained a great deal of confidence in myself and I know from the things we went through I can and will not roll in pity."

Setbacks occur because we may have lost sight of what is within our limits. I may have to discern where and when to detach. If I detach in the process of taking care of myself I will still be sad over this detachment. If there was an involvement to begin with there is probably caring for this person, to detach will bring sadness. I setback because I allowed myself to feel negative about a recent detachment. I had forgotten it is normal to feel sad when we experience a loss. The loss was not my fault. My loss was due to the misperceptions of another. I had to detach. Detach in level three. I believe there are three levels of detachment. They are;

1. In our head we know it is their shortcoming that has created a problem but we feel, if I do ...... it might help.

2. I now know the problem is due to their shortcoming. I have learned what control is and isn't . I have learned that I have taken responsibility for their actions by thinking what I could do would fix a situation. I now tell myself the thing I want to do is control. I don't do it. But I want to. I have learned not to move in with a fix but I still want to fix.

3. The best and final level of detachment has come our way. We detach from a person or situation because we know it is what is best for us. We have no guilt for taking care of ourselves. We don't even think about reacting in controlling ways. We don't fix nor do we want to fix. We have come to feel peace of mind with the heart felt knowledge of how good it is not to fix.

My setbacks come about when I am not able to stay in level three. I may regress to level two. I may ponder over why I wish to control. I may hit the pits of level one or go all the way back to taking the blame for their wrongdoing.

I came to understand normal, functional people, have negative times and feelings. The sooner I can tell myself and believe everyone has setbacks the sooner I am able to think positive. The sooner I am able to think positive the faster I am able to pull myself together. Think positive. Do what I need to do to take care of my thoughts and feelings. In reality, I am the only one that is responsible to see to it that I am happy. Peter Pans trick was, "it only takes one happy thought," and he could fly. If I am able to think one positive, happy thought I am able to get my line of cognitive thinking in motion. I can fly. I stop, ask my God, "give me one positive thought, give me the strength to take it from there." He always does. End to setback.

When I don't know where I go from here it is time to look at my negative thoughts and see how I can benefit from them. Benefit from negative thoughts and feelings. I can take a look and find out why I feel negative. This may lead to a new discovery on my part. The things I need to know are calling to me. They will point the way. This will lead to positive thinking as I learn the lesson I need to know to successfully continue with my life.

"I need my feelings even if they are negative. I still need them. If only to remind myself that I am not perfect. If only to enjoy the beauty of my averageness. I cannot do everything right. I don't do everything wrong. I like me even though I can't do everything right. I love me even though I can't do everything right. I feel good about myself. I am not arrogant for thinking and feeling that I am a person worth knowing.

When I have negative feelings about myself I can use those negative feelings to grow. I can let them remind me of the importance of staying on the road of recovery. Let us never assume we are fully recovered lest we slip back into the old dysfunctional patterns of behavior. My occasional negative thoughts can help me to realize how important it is to enforce my boundaries, to properly separate baggage and to acknowledge my limits. My negative feeling can work for me like a radar detector and tell me where and when to slow down and take a careful look at what I am doing. See my mistake and get back on track. I have accepted I am normal. I am average. I am human. I am me." from A JOURNAL OF GROWTH, A WORKBOOK.

It was the above quote that inspired me to write this section in this book. I could look back at what I wrote during a setback and grow. I took strength from the negative thoughts I had experienced at that time. I can draw strength from positive thoughts and actions of others or myself. I can draw strength from the negative thoughts and actions of others. I can identify where I used to be and where I am today.

We introduced this section talking about the benefits of writing. Write the negative. Write the positive. Refer back to them from time to time. Draw on and grow from the positive. Draw on and grow from the negative. When I am able to analyze the negative, feel what I must feel about the negative and turn it over, use it for positive growth I am learning the true art of recovery. I am learning I need not downward spiral in times of setback. I am learning to use a setback not to setback yet more but to see the lesson I need to know, use the wisdom I have learned, apply my new knowledge in my life, and continue to heal from dysfunction.

Keep in mind when we are in a time of setback we will not perform verbal judo appropriately. We will not communicate as accurately as we have learned. We will not fight with dignity as well or as often. Our self esteem will lack the degree we have achieved. We probably will say many wrong things to co-workers, spouses, and our beloved children. This is why it is a setback, it is not a backforever. Muster strength by doing the things we know work for us. Tell our children the parts that are our fault. Grow together. Functional does not mean we do this 100% 100% of the time. We can model to our family, our next generation, our function, an approving attitude of ourselves and of them when we are not able to do as well as at other times. We need not be perfect to be okay. This is the true art of being functional. This is the true process of breaking the cycle of abuse.

SADNESS, DEPRESSION AND GETTING BETTER

Sadness is a normal emotion. Sadness is the strength to accept negative situations without allowing the negative situation to reflect on our level of self esteem. Sadness is a natural response to look at any situation realistically. We accept our loss or disappointment in an undistorted way.

Depression on the other hand is always a result from distorted thoughts. Either depression or sadness can develop after a loss or a failure to reach a desired goal. One that was of great importance to us. Sadness comes without any distortion. Our feelings flow through us. It has a time limit. We grieve our loss or losses a degree at a time until not only our mind but our heart and soul have released the pain resulting from the loss. At this time we are able to accept in our heart the value of whatever gains have come to us as a result of this negative situation. My gain may be empathy for others in a subject area I knew nothing of prior to this time. My gain may be something new to me that will directly affect my life and my person. Sadness has helped me to move on with my life a degree at a time. I have not lost my self esteem. I can be sad without taking the blame for my mistakes and the mistakes of others. Learning this was a great mental boost to me. I thought that I had fought depression most of my life. In reality much of what I thought was depression was sadness. I had been fighting against sadness. Doing whatever it took to block out my sadness. Is it any wonder the day would come when I would hobble through my front door broken foot and all and the next thing I knew I was fetal position on the floor screaming, "I can't take anymore. No more! No more!" From that point I started to improve. I little here and there. It would, however, be a year later before I would enter therapy. After being in therapy about a year I began to read Feeling Good by Dr. David Burns. In the front of his book there is a small test to evaluate the extent of depression. I took this test trying to relate to the questions as to how I felt when I entered therapy. I venture to say if I had told my therapist the extent of my feelings I would have been hospitalized. I, in my dysfunction, had learned not to reveal too much. I had begun to speak about the things that had hurt me and created my dysfunction. I had begun to see how the things I did continued my dysfunction. I had also learned to give myself credit for the changes I had made over the years. I had not learned to trust enough to tell how badly I really felt. All part of my depression, all part of my, I'm not doing this good enough, all part of my be strong at all cost. Then I learned that sadness is the strength to accept our circumstances for what they really are. The ability to look at the bad as well as the good. Now I could grieve what I needed to grieve, feel what I needed to feel, express to certain others what I feel and felt, and still know I was and am not weak, I was and am strong. I do have the strength to accept my realities. I do have the strength to be sad. My favorite way of expressing my ability to accept sadness and know my strength is summed up in the next statement. **Strong means, I do what I have to do to handle my life. I can cry while I do it. If I want to**.

With depression our feelings are frozen. We lock them inside of ourselves. Our self esteem is the main target of our depression. Arrows of negativity head for our target, hit the bulls eye and we collapse, degrade ourselves, get involved in compulsive behaviors, don't know what is wrong with us, blame others for our problems, wrap ourselves in a cloak of distorted thinking. Statements like, "I can never be happy without him," demonstrate our inability to be complete from within ourselves. We have frozen into unhappiness. We expect to be unhappy. We get what we expect. With unhappiness we lose even more self esteem. Without self esteem we are unable or unwilling to establish or enforce our boundaries. Establishing and enforcing our boundary or mistake or if it is pointed out to us we take responsibility for our flaws. We can readjust a boundary if we find it inappropriate. If the other person still rejects us it is their lack of empathy, their dysfunctional thinking that brings about their rejection of us. We need not take it personal. We need not target in on our self esteem creating a cycle of depression and dysfunction. We can be sad because of someone else's rejection. We need not become depressed over it. I can know I am good enough. I do handle this situation or problem in the way I honestly feel is most appropriate. I know I have evaluated how I feel about the situation, taken an honest look at the positives and the negatives. How I handle it may not be the same as how you handle it. I am however good enough. I have now accepted my feelings without digging into depression. I am enhancing my self esteem even when I am sad. Enforcing our boundaries is a key ingredient to being able to accept sadness while at the same time realizing that I am not having a setback because I am sad. With that in view I would like to say:

I am not having a setback when I feel sad.
I am not experiencing setback when I am mad.
Any feeling that I feel,
Is human, normal, and very real.

If I believe setback this makes
I not likely to have what it takes
to face my realities
with a smile or a tear
to be able to say
life do come here.

Whatever feeling that I do feel
is normal, natural, and real.
When this truth I know from my heart
my self esteem from me not departs.

To have my boundaries
to be able to say,
"I feel sad,"
is one of the greatest joys that can be had.

It took me a while to associate in my mind the truth about setbacks.

I am not having a setback when I'm sad.
I am not having a setback when I am mad.
I am not having a setback when I don't know what to do.
I am not having a setback when I realize a limit (something I can not do).

These all I consider crucial to the subject of sadness verses depression. In my dysfunction negative feelings were the things I blocked out, denied. As I learned how to face my feelings I was very upset to find out how often I had anger. "That's not me." I said. Every time I had anger or sadness I felt like, "what's wrong with me?" Why? Because I was not used to accepting anger or sadness. I had learned not to deny I had them but it would take time before I made the connection that whenever I was feeling these things I was not having a setback. I believe if I allow these things to tell me I am not doing this good enough, I don't know what's wrong with me, then my level of self esteem is being affected, then I am having a setback. One day, when angry, I blurted out, "I'm not having a setback because I'm angry. You would be angry too if...." this brought about a whole new realization. Since that time I no longer have depression, even if short lived (several minutes), over whatever emotion I am feeling. I am able to acknowledge my feeling, know I know appropriate ways to handle this feeling, know ways to take care of myself without hurting others, and relax. I am not depressed. I can now enforce my boundaries and still be considerate of the other person. I can establish, build, and hold on to a healthy relationship, if that is what we both desire. A healthy relationship is one where both parties are willing to consider the boundaries, self esteem issues and rights, of the other person. A healthy relationship is one where both parties are willing to flex without stepping on the other person's boundaries or forsaking their boundaries. Being able to live these principles allows us to become more functional. The more functional we are the more confident we become. The more confident we become the more functional we are, another paradox. The more functional we are the better able we are to accept sadness, know we have validate reasons for our sadness, know that our sadness does not fault us as a person. Concerning boundaries and limits I said, "I can't do this." My counselor said, "You are doing it, you have been doing it." Simple? Yes, but true. I was doing it. It felt better and better each time I practiced or carried out my new found skills. Each time I stood for what I said some of my fear dissipated. Yes, I was nervous. I tried my best not to let on. I continued to practice applying my boundaries. It worked. It is now the joy of my life to know I can take care of me without hurting you. Each time I practice appropriately enforcing my boundaries I have less cause to be sad. I do not allow myself to be used. I now feel the genuine feeling of happiness. The relationships I have are truly relationships. I help where I want to help. If I begin to feel used I say, "I need to tell you how I feel about this situation." If I feel the other party is not approachable at that time I ask myself, "What is it I need to change to deal with this situation?" or "Do I need to walk away or do I need to wait for a more appropriate time to talk to them? Do I feel that talking to this person will make any difference in this situation? If not maybe I need to withdraw my help." When doing any or all of the above I am taking care of myself and eliminating many causes of sadness. This does not mean that I will never feel sadness. When I do I have the ability to be sad and accept my strengths all at the same time.

Reactive depression is a depression that comes from obvious stress. The death of a loved one, a business reversal and/or bad health. When we are sick we cannot do the things we did. We can easily become depressed. All of us need to feel the things we do make a difference in this world. When we cannot do, a natural reaction is to reflect on our value as a person. We are also measuring our worth by the things we do. Do we measure the worth of other people by what they do? If that were the case why do we so highly value the life of a babe? But value them we do. Why should I now judge myself differently than I do others? I can be tolerant and supportive to others and to myself. Am I understanding when someone else is not able to live up to what they promised me and harsh on myself when I am not able to do something that I had set as a goal? Realistically dealing with my sickness and the sadness that will result from not being able to do what I want and feel I need to do means that I feel sadness because I cannot do what I prefer to do. Preferring to do and having to do to prove my worth are two different stories. I need not have two sets of standards. One for others and a harsher, intolerant one for myself. Apply the same rules to myself as I kindly extend to others. If I don't feel their mistakes or lack of ability to do make them bad or worthless than why would I be bad or worthless? All or nothing thinking paralyzes us into fear of failure, perhaps fear of even trying.

When my daughter was sixteen I gave her some very bad advice. She was old enough to start working and wanted a part time job after school. My boss said he would love to have her work for him. She said, "I don't want to live in you shadow mom." She went on to express how she was not near as capable as I. I told her that was not the case. "You, my dear, are better at different things than I am. You see what I do. I just do the things that I do well. You don't have to mention the things you can't do. No one will know but you. Everyone tells me how capable I am. That is because all they see is what I do well. I can't knit. You can. I can't sew very well, you can. So do what you do well and don't worry about other things. Take pride in the things you are good at."

If I had to give advice to her today I would say that only the last sentence of the above quote is worth paying attention to. I would add to it not to be afraid to try new things. If you fail or are only average, so what. We cannot excel at everything and I need not ignore the things I do not do well. My art work looks like a third graders. If I was called upon to illustrate this book we could all laugh about it, even me, especially me.

We have been sad or depressed for a long time. It is time to get better.

FEELING BETTER OR GETTING BETTER

Feeling better and getting better are two different things. I had several periods of serious depression that I managed to get through but I was not better. I had not resolved the causes of my depression. I thought that the things others, I love, did were the cause of my depression. I thought, we all have times that are good and times that are bad and since we are not perfect we will have disappointments with ourselves and with others. When that happens we need to get through it however we can. I always had. "I'm better now," I'd say. I needed to find the causes of my sadness and depression, finish my business. I had been treating the symptoms and not the cause. I would come to liken it to chopping a weed off at the ground. If we take care of the real problem we will dig up the roots, however hard it may be, throw the whole thing away. No more chopping it off at the ground. No more depression.

Dr. David Burns in his book FEELING GOOD discusses getting better by finding the cause. To paraphrase Dr. Burns we must:

1. Know why we became depressed.

2. Know how and why we got better. We must master the skills that have helped us. We must have wisdom, the ability to use the things we have learned in new and different situations that arise in our life in the present. The problems I have now in my life are lessen not by denial, not by minimization, but by my ability to use my functionality. Functionality is my ability to use the things I learned in whatever life brings my way. I need not go to therapy or a group all my life. I go to therapy or groups long enough to learn basic principles and then a fine tuning process. I now am functional. I know how and why I got better. At one point I became seriously overwhelmed by information that came my way without my looking for it. This information cast a whole new light on subjects and individuals I thought were settled. I was tossed and turned but my anchor was secure. During the tossing process I didn't feel secure. I learned that I as a functional person I will feel tossed about from time to time but I do know what the problem is. I didn't and don't have guilt for any of the things I needed to feel to get myself back on track. I said at that time, "I don't know what to do." The reply was, "Yes you do, you do all

the same things you did in your original therapy." My mind gave way to an, "OH, NO! NOT AGAIN!" But I did them. I talked. I cried. I wrote. I realized why I felt so betrayed. I could examine the whole gambit of ambivalent feelings I had. I felt anger, sadness, confusion, ambivalence, resentment, betrayal, fear, hurt, and soon I would come to feel relief, safe, joy, and peace of mind. Peace from knowing the truth. I ran the gambit of feelings all humans feel. I had learned however to use each feeling for my best benefit. Only a short time in the beginning of this ordeal did I relapse into depression. I allowed what others were saying about me in different subject areas to add to the burden of what I already must sort. I felt weak, drained, sad, and added to my burden by allowing myself to be put down by the verbal abuse of others.

Today as I write I am sorting and using the things I learned in my process of learning how to act in a functional way. I am as I write feeling the joy of knowing that an extremely difficult situation, an on going situation, one I have had to accept with pain in my heart, one that will not change, moves me to tears, is being handled by myself and other family members in such a way that I know that without my recovery process this situation would have driven me to therapy. This situation could have driven my entire family apart. This has not been the case. Our family has bonded, talked, sorted, and united their souls becoming more functional with each distress. This is only so because I know how and why I got better. I use, role model (a[illegible] step twelve) the joy of recovery. This is how I stay recovered. This is how I stay functional. This is how my family is growing in their function.

3. Acknowledge our current level of self esteem. Acknowledge the hard work we have done. This is apply part two. We know how we got where we are today as regards our self esteem. We are aware of the effects and affects of slipping self esteem. We also are aware of the steps we can take to resort our self esteem. We have made personal relationships work, we have made successes of careers we only dream of prior to this time. We have come to love ourselves for what we are not what we wish to be. We are what we wish to be. The things I do not like about myself I acknowledge to myself and others when appropriate without shame or guilt, knowing I will work to improve where I can.

4. We have found the deeper causes of our depression. We finished our business. Released much of our sadness. Learn how to address any feelings we have as soon as we are aware of them.

A great deal of our sadness was created by us as we set standards that were so high that it truly amazes me how we ever accomplished anything. Frustration was the name of the game. Dysfunction breeds frustration. Frustration allows us to be in the control of others who like to verbally abuse, criticize, and deride. My frustration with myself made me an open target for the verbally aggressive. I thought that none of us see ourselves as others see us so when others criticized me I felt there was a good chance they might be right since I may be inclined to overlook my faults. Now, I look over my faults. Take another look. Examine myself for myself. I can listen to the criticism of others as long as they attempt to state their feelings in a respectful way. To the verbally aggressive I say, "I am willing to listen to what you have to say if we can sit down and discuss this in a rational way." To those that continue to be verbally aggressive I have said, "I feel this may not be the best time. Can we talk about this tomorrow?" or I have said, "Excuse me, if we can clam down I will be glad to talk with you if that is not the case I will leave." This is seldom necessary. But to the verbally abusive my boundary is stated and applied for my continued ability to act in a functional way. (In other words so when they blow their cool I will not blow my cool simply because I failed to enforce my right not to be verbally abused). Also stated as the following; **I will lose my cool if I listen to you losing your cool long enough.**

My continued state of internal sadness, regardless of how competent or together I looked on the outside, left me with the perpetual and awful feeling that I could not be alone. This led me to make several very bad decisions. Two of the most common bad decisions of all womanhood. First my choice of a marriage mate. Second my decision or basic lack of decision to care for myself after I was in the marriage. My worst decision was to stay in that marriage. A violent, abusive nonrelationship that almost cost me my life. This I perceived as better than being alone. I thought that being alone would be the worst thing that could happen to me. No one to love me. No one to care about if I exist. I almost died. I had to suffer broken ribs, a broken jaw and internal damage that would take it's toll as years went on before I would leave that marriage. I left in fear. An arsenal of guns in the truck of his car and the basement of our home as well as bows and arrows in the hands of a master shot caused me to leave with my children in fear of our lives.

I came to see how wrong I had been. I became a single parent of two preschoolers. I took care of my children and lived my life knowing my bills were paid, not having to worry about where the money would be blown this week. I came to feel happy to be alone with my children. I could do a few things like I wanted. I could come and go from my own home and not worry what would happen as I walked through the door. I was learning how to take responsibility for my own life.

As I wrote the paragraph stating why I stayed in such a dangerous marriage I laughed and said to my husband (different husband) "Was I sick?" He raised his eyebrows. I said, "You don't even have to answer. I WAS SICK."

Our negative self image is a self defeating image or system. We can not only feel better we can get better. We can discover and work through the reasons for our dysfunction, chronic low self esteem, and depression. Our negative self image remains constant whether we are depressed or in remission. It has been said that low self esteem is another term for being approval addicted, love addicted and achievement addicted. My dysfunction led me to believe that I could not function without love from another of the male gender. From this I thought I would get approval, love, a sense of purpose, fulfillment, and a sense of completeness. Being alone left me knowing how incomplete I was. Being with another allowed me to concentrate on their problems, not my incompleteness.

I needed to reassess my standards. I needed to realize that just because I felt I was entitled did not mean that I would get what I felt entitled to. We are imperfect people in an imperfect world. We will get what we are entitled to when the world is perfect. I wanted respect. Am I entitled? Yes. Does that mean I will get respect from others? No. If I conduct my life in a respectful way than I will probably be respected by some. That does not mean they will tell me about it. Others will not respect my level of function. Some will feel intimidated by my functionality. The greater their dysfunction the more they will be intimidated by my function. We cannot demand their respect. Their dysfunction has left them in a state of confusion about the changes we have made. For this they give not respect. I came to be able to detach from how they perceived my changes. Some of the people I felt I needed respect from did not act in a respectful way. I felt like, "What was it all for? I worked so hard to break the cycle only to watch as the cycle starts over again. Let go. Let go of control. What was it all for?" I now know. It was for me. I am not depressed. I have joy of heart and peace of mind. I am not afraid of being alone. I found my true complete self, the child that hid. She only hid. She was not lost. She was not crushed or destroyed. She only hid, hoping one day to be found, allowing herself to be found. She was watching from inside of me. Waiting for recognition. She finally got my attention. I would like to think that somewhere down the line someone will remember, someone healed. They can do it when they want.

Our healing, our moving on to being functional from dysfunction is our process of gaining autonomy. Autonomy is the ability to find happiness within ourselves. If we wait for external forces to make us happy it will not happen. I think a vital point to remember is that external forces can make us happy for moments, days, or weeks, but when a negative external force joins in we are stripped of whatever happiness we gained from the positive external forces. This happiness would be better called a mood. Mood is defined by Webster as 1. a particular state of mind or feeling; humor or temper. 2. a prevailing feeling, spirit, or tone. 3. fits of morose (ill tempered, characterized by gloom), sullen, or uncertain temper. By definition we see an overall prevailing sense of gloom. This I think tempers the word mood accurately. We say we are in a good mood. The mood however is controlled by external forces which knowing the realities of life can turn negative in a second. Joy is the true condition of the heart. We can have joy and be sad at the same time when we are complete. Our joy is knowing who we are, what makes us tick, how to disprove an attitude, our joy is the foundation of our autonomy. We can be who and what we are as we do not fear being rejected by others. We do not need to please others to feel approved. I feel approved from myself. I need the approval of only two persons in this universe. Myself and my God. I live my life in the way I know he will approve. He has not left mankind in the dark. Through His word he gave to all of us an outline of the type of faith and actions he requires. Within this framework millions of people have come to have his approval, each and every one of them different from another. He does not care if we are fat or thin, black or white or brown or red, he does not care what our preference of decor, dress, food, or mannerism are. None of the above reflect on the quality of our person. They do reflect on the style of our person not the quality. All these joys are mine as I become autonomous. The freedom to be myself without fear of what others may think about what I think. Without fear of jumping to conclusions about what others think. Life is not a burden. It has become a thrill.

My autonomy allows me to act legitimate, original. I am no longer outerdirected. I have no control over almost everything in this universe. If I allow external forces to control my actions I am being controlled. I give up their control of me by examining my beliefs. I must decide what I believe, why I believe it, and whether or not it is in my best interest to keep believing this. I can assess my beliefs in the light of the evidence. The evidence is the results that have come from my belief. If I believe that I am inadequate because I made a mistake then in turn I feel more inadequate. My belief has generated itself, also called a self fulfilling prophecy. Fear of failure or inadequacy has recycled itself, proving or seeming to prove itself to be true. Cognitive thinking tells us to put this belief to the test. If I believe I am inadequate and I make a mistake I can try again. This time I succeed. I have proved my mistaken belief just that, mistaken. If I fail again I can think of things I do right. Just because I fail at one thing does not mean I fail at everything. My husband is a chemist. I almost failed chemistry. I wrote a book. My husband almost failed English. We are each successes in our own right.

Dr. David Burns in his book FEELING GOOD shows us how we can go about finding what he calls the path of independence and self respect. We do a cost benefit analysis. Businesses do this before undertaking a project. Is it worth the risk? We weight the advantages against the disadvantages of letting others determine our worth. List the ways this hurts and helps us. We will probably find that it hurts us more that it helps us. Is the keeping of this rule, belief, to our advantage or best interest. I think not. Rewrite the rule. Record over old tapes. Maybe throw it away entirely. I changed my, "I need their approval," thought or rule to "I don't need their approval. It would be nice to have it, but I don't need it." Whether it is nice to have their approval or not depends on the price we have to pay. My price had been dysfunction. Not needing their approval gave my life a new and better purpose, a new and better meaning. I can be the unique and precious person I was born to be.

Why do we get so upset when someone disapproves of us? We conclude this must mean that others will also disapprove. When we are complimented it doesn't make us feel good unless we belief the compliment. The same is true about insults. If we believe them our mood reflects them. We have paid a high price for their approval. We have forsaken us. The opinions of others make or break us. We set ourselves up to be abandoned again and again. If we don't buy it it cannot control us.

Their disapproval is their problem. Their lack of empathy, their irrational thoughts, is their problem. If we find we have made a serious mistake that may have jeopardized this relationship we can do steps 8 and 9 of any twelve step program. Step eight is to be willing to make amends, then when the time feels right to approach the other person or persons and make amends where possible for whatever my part in the situation was. And I would add I base this decision on having prayed about the matter, asking for wisdom to see my shortcomings and to let me know what it is I need to do and to use good sense in my timing with each of the things I do. I can allow them to express how they feel about what happened. Here comes an important boundary of mine. I will listen as someone points out a flaw of mine. This I do because I cannot realistically see all my flaws. Their words could be the vehicle used by my God to give me the information for which I asked. If however they begin to harangue me over my wrong doing, if I feel this is turning into their opportunity to verbal abuse me for my error I state, "I came here to make amends for the wrong I did. I sincerely regret this. I do not feel that I need to be put down because of what I did. I know my wrong that is why I am here to make amends." That is my more tactful version to an upset person. To myself I state: **"I came here to make amends. I will not allow you to verbally abuse me for the thing I am attempting to make amends for."**

When I offer amends I allow them to disapprove of the thing I did. This does not mean they disapprove of me. All of us at some time or another have said unkind, hurtful things to people we love. We have made it clear how strongly we disapprove of their thoughts and/or actions. We choose not to associate with some because we do not agree with their behavior. We even told them of our low opinion of their behavior. Does that make them, "no good," absolutely, "no good." I don't believe so. We may come to regret what we said. It may be totally untrue. If it is true or even partly true it still does not prove their total worthlessness. If that is true when we do it to others cognitive thinking would tell us it is true when others do it to us. Why give others the power to devaluate us. If and when others point out our faults we can listen. Think about what they said. See if we do it. If we conclude that we do then we can make appropriate changes. We can learn and grow. Grow more functional. Break the cycle of dysfunction. We are breaking the cycle of blaming ourselves for the thoughts and actions of others.

I find that every aspect of recovery from dysfunction is interwoven with every other aspect. As we break the cycle of dysfunction we establish boundaries. We learn to communicate boundaries to others. We learn to change boundaries when necessary without feeling we will not be taken seriously. We learn to detach from the negative perceptions of others. The more we are able to detach from the thoughts and feelings of others the better we will be at setting and enforcing our boundaries. Here we are back to our earlier discussion of how the better we enforce our boundaries the less sadness we have. Our boundaries are our way of saying this is what can and can't be done here. If I allow you to..... around me or in my house than I feel used.

"In order to make and enforce my boundaries, I do have to assess the situation as realistically as possible considering the facts that I know. If I ask others for feedback or information about the circumstances that we hopefully will deal with together and they lie or manipulate me, I can only do the best that I can.

I believe when I like myself, when I respect myself, when I quit expecting me to get everything right, when I accept my limits (at least most of the time), when boundaries are easier to enforce than deny my right to have them, when I am not afraid of detachment (I know that my boundaries may cost me a relationship and I still stand by my boundary in order to take care of my feelings), when I am doing all these things because I need to care and take care of myself, then I am not," dysfunctional. Quoted for Journal of Growth, A Workbook.

In order to not allow sadness to rule and ruin my life I must detach. Others who disapproved of me made clear to me their disapproval and why. I really hurt. I knew I had to detach in order to heal, to grow more functional. Being functional became everything to me. It is what I had been looking for all my life. The joy of accurate communication especially under difficult circumstances. The joy of knowing many difficult circumstances are prevented by accurate communication while the problem is small. In working through our dysfunction we are laying a new foundation for a new relationship, new ground rules. When we detached from certain others we both believed our losses were permanent. This is hardly ever true. Most people want to keep important relationships important. We can both adjust to the new ground rules. This is especially true when the relationship is between parents and their children. The children may be adults but that does not change the fact that not many people are capable of totally writing off a parent or their child, adult or not, and never seeing or speaking again. My boundary in this situation is: I am an adult. I am a grandma of five. To my parents I say, "Let's talk about this as three adults that we are. We can agree to disagree without faulting another." At one time I needed to say, "I am an adult. I will listen to you as long as you speak to me as an adult not as the child I once was. I was your child. Now I am an adult who prefers to have a relationship with parents that respect my adulthood. I will not criticize you if you think and feel different than I. What I want back from you is the same. This I feel is the true meaning of respect. So if we need to talk, let's."

In some cases this boundary will not be respected. If we need to detach we will feel sad. This is normal. We need not turn our sadness into depression. Sadness does not reflect on our self worth. Well, maybe it does. My ability to accept my sadness, to know my strength through my sadness has allowed me to become the real self that I am. Grieving what I needed to grieve released pain and sorrow, stress and anxiety from my heart and from my literal body. No more insomnia. No more indigestion, no more anxiety attacks. Seldom do I have a headache and when I do I identify what the cause. Almost always I have pushed my limits. I have overworked. This too has allowed me to learn about myself. When I overwork it is always in connection with writing, publishing, and distributing. Why did I overwork? Because I love to write. I like many of the things I have learned about myself through publishing and distributing. I have learning I am a very creative person. This I did not know. When I was dysfunctional my style of getting approval, being good enough, was to work very hard. If I do this I will be good enough. Today I have learned about myself that I overwork because I love this kind of work. I like being alone. I like being at my computer seeing words, thoughts, and ideas being expressed on my computer screen. Knowing they will turn into manuscript and then into a book. A book that can be read by any who choose. A book that may contain a thought of two that help another. This is my way of working step twelve. To spread the good news of healing to others. I have learned about myself through my writing, through my overdoing my limits at times that I have healed from the need of approval. I do none of these things because I need to to be okay. I do them because it gives me joy of heart. This is a process that allows me to be me. At one time I said, "I don't know what difference it makes if I put words down on paper or not." But it does. This is me. This is what makes me tick. Communication that I longed for all my life is at my fingertips. I can communicate with myself, my loved ones (no matter the circumstances) and through the pages of my books I can communicate with the world.

BEING ALONE OR BEING LONELY

Loneliness could best be described as a heavy stone in our heart. Loneliness leaves us empty and full of despair. Loneliness leaves us feeling we have no connection to the rest of the world, like a motherless child, small--lost in a vast uncaring world. As I read the words motherless child I felt the vastness of the loneliness I had lived with much of my life.

To be lonely means to be isolated from ourself. To be alone is to have time by myself to get to know the real me in an intimate way. Enjoy being with myself. This is a true joy I have attained in recent years. I love to be home alone in the quietness of my house type on a book, read a book, sort my thoughts. No back ground music, no people talking, just me. I can and do take time to think and feel what I need to think and feel. I can take to mediate. Time to sort and separate. Reflect on my feelings, use what I learn to grow. Time not to think about anything is another luxury I give to myself. Time to unwind. Relax.

I can keep myself so busy I don't think about what I think or how I feel. This is a form of denial. A way to say, "I am good enough because I am important to all these people and all these projects." If I am afraid to not be busy or afraid to be alone with myself I am lonely. I isolate myself from others by staying so busy with projects that I don't have time for relationships I am dysfunctional. Dysfunction basically is someone who is so caught up in the whatever they do not function in the day in day out relationships with other people. If I have never taken the time to be alone with myself, know myself how will I be able to know another.

For many years I struggled with the concept of how to disprove an attitude. The answer is simple. I must look inside of me. I can come to know what makes me tick. When I was in sixth grade my teacher taught me to diagram sentences and by the end of the year he told me that he had taught me all he knew about English and he had a masters degree in English. True enough I could diagram compound complex sentences without a moments hesitation but I had not learned to use those same skills of observation, the skills involved in the mechanics of the inner workings of myself, to break down the different elements of me, to find what makes me tick, to disprove an attitude. I entered therapy when I was forty years old and I learned how to diagram myself. How to look inside of me and say, "This is my dangling participle, this is the conjunction I need to make these two pieces fit, this is the adverb that best describes what I felt when, all the inner workings put together in the most difficult sentence in the world to diagram. Yes, I could diagram any sentence in the world except one, the one I came to understand, comprehend and diagram with peace of mind and joy of heart. The most difficult sentence in the world to diagram. What was it?------- Who am I? The New York Times Magazine of April 28, 1991 stated about the pain of lonely children, their pain was the pain of, "the wounds of friendlessness." I enjoy writing. One of the most flattering compliments I have received was just the other day from a woman that has read most of my books. Upon meeting she said, "As I read your books I have to say that I felt that Dee Frances would just explode if she could not write." We laughed. "You're right. I suppose I would." I believe it is therefore safe to say, "I love writing." I do my best when I am alone. I am not lonely. I feel genuinely fulfilled and nurtured. Writing provides to me the channel I need to sort feelings, to look at things realistically, and to remind myself of things forgotten, helpful positive thoughts I had long forgotten. As I write I find fulfillment in renewing what I have forgotten and joy in researching for information to expand on what I know. Weaving them together like a priceless tapestry as the words of this page appear. As I weave the information together I know what I am learning I then connect it with how I can use these particular thoughts, feelings, ideas, philosophies in my life and my circumstances. I also consider others who have spoken with me and their attitudes and preferences and I, at times, make notes to give to them on thoughts they may like whether or not they are applicable to myself. I believe I am at my best when I write. I touch my inner core, the heart of my soul, exposing it for all the world to see without fear of being judged adversely if those who read this book happen to disagree with some of it's contents. What I think and feel on paper for all to see. How's that for a former dysfunctional person.

Am I lonely? On the contrary, I am happy, fulfilled, gratified, pleased with myself, growing, adjusting, enthusiastic and learning. I am writing and through my writing I am accomplishing a life long dream.

I believe our purpose for being is to love and to be loved? Am I needing other peoples approval to accomplish this? I don't believe so. I love myself. I had to learn the process of letting go of pains of the past one degree at a time in order to forgive myself for my wrongs as well as my supposed wrongs. I came to learn the process of forgiving myself with which came love for myself. I am loved. Loved by myself and another important other. He loves us all in spite of what we do. He does not like many of the things we do. He is always there for us. John 3:16 "God loved the world so much...." The Greek word for world is kosmos. In English we derive the word cosmopolitan from the Greek, Kosmos. Cosmopolitan refers to groups of people. So at John 3: 16 it is not saying God loved the planet earth so much. It is saying God loved the world of mankind so much. If I never have acceptance from other humans my purpose to love and be loved can still be fulfilled. I can have the approval of the two most important persons, my God and myself. I am never really alone.

When my youngest child started school I was at loose ends. I had taken care of children since I was five, I had taken care of and taken responsibility for siblings older than myself, and now I found myself alone. What would I do with myself? I was nervous and afraid. My baby was in school and I, his mother, had reached a turning point in my life. It didn't take long for me to realize how much I liked the quite. I finally had time to think. Time for me. The many years of hearing Big Bird in the background were gone. What a relief! I could probably site the dialogues by heart. Time to sit and read a book, time to reflect, time to work toward some of the goals I wanted. I started to know myself for the first time. I did not always like what I discovered but I had time to study and learn. I started working in areas of special interest to me. The void, the knot in my gut, or the hole in my soul was closing. I had started giving to others not because I felt compelled but because this is what I genuinely wanted to do. Soon the hole in my gut had vanished, giving to others in a truly spiritual way closed the hole in my soul, the knot in my gut was gone. Other things which had previously taken my time, things that my dysfunction had caused me to do, became less and less a part of my life. I simply did not have time to do everything I did and the new things I wanted to do. I was starting to realize, I can't do it all, some things are more important than others. This is my list of things to do, in order of my priorities. I will do as much as I can but I, too, have limits. I, too, get tired. I still, however, drove myself. While I prioritized my list I still had a do tomorrow list. I had let up to some extent but still expected too much in too little time. I had though started the process of letting go. I worked until I was exhausted. As time went by I became more balanced about what my limits are, less and less influenced by the dysfunctional thinking of others and/or myself.

Eight years ago I could not watch a television show without doing something else at the same time. I would mend, iron, write bills, write letters, anything that would say to me, "It's okay to sit down. You are not wasting time. You are being productive." Six years ago I started slowing down but to compensate for my guilt while I did I'd say, "I get tired too. I think I'm entitled." Today, I take a break whenever I feel the need. After a short break I can return to whatever, if I choose. I have found I am more productive but on the occasions where I am not I do not feel bad, guilty, or lazy. I have taken the time to acknowledge I, as a person, have needs. Many of those needs will be expressed by and through my limitations. I have discovered I am not only okay I am a person worth knowing. I always wanted to live my life in a way that it would have made a worth while difference that I was here. I have come to realize, "I have."

My husband took our son up to his college campus. I stayed home to work on a book. I came to the point of needing a break. I went to a movie, alone. This was a first. It was also nice. I am not lonely under any circumstances nor am I isolated from myself. I connect. I connect not only with others I connect with myself and the universe.

Our dysfunction can be triggered by circumstances in the present which are entirely different than the circumstances of our past, circumstances however, which create the same type of feelings within us conjuring up the same type of rejection and pain. If we felt rejected by a certain person or set of circumstances then in other circumstances where we feel rejected we have revisited our old circumstances and also have the present circumstances with which to deal. Think about what is going on with ourselves. What is a common thread. For me, a common thread amounted to personal losses. I wanted to have my gains without any losses. Reality does not work in that way. For every gain we will have a loss, unfortunately some of our losses will be people. People we may love. Our loss will bring pain, with the pain of their loss will also come the joy of one less dysfunctional nonrelationship.

I have come to understand, I can only be abandoned when I abandon myself. If I need other peoples approval to be okay I am lonely, isolated from myself. Once I approve of, validate me, meaning my feelings are valid (important) I never need be lonely again. The things I do by myself can be just as satisfying as the things I do with others. We typically plan activities with other people. Sometimes things are as much fun as we thought they would be, other times they are not. That's life. So be it when we are alone. If something turns out not to be what we had anticipated we need not connect this with the fact we were alone. When we do not have as much fun out of something we do with other people we do not say, "well, I'll never go any where with other people again" If going by ourself is a bit upsetting make it a goal to be less uncomfortable with each endeavor. Jeffrey Young commented in September 17, 1984 U.S. News & World Report, "Some lonely people....turn potential friends off, either by monopolizing the discussion or by saying things that are obnoxious or inappropriate. One way or another, chronically lonely people tend to sabotage close relationships."

Our thoughts produce our feelings. How we think about any circumstance determines how we feel. Thoughts, the most powerful things in the universe, control us. If we think negative we will be negative. If we think being alone means being lonely we will be lonely. Research has proven that writing out our thoughts is part of any healing process. Our own personal experience shows that we can speed our healing. We can sort and separate our thoughts and feelings from the events in our life. As we start to write our real feelings begin to surface, feelings we may not have been aware we had. In his book FEELING GOOD Dr. David Burns outlines many different writing exercises we can do. Each of which help us to find the source of a problem. Each of which help us to compare our distorted thinking to more rational ways of thinking. Such as, "I am unhappy because I am alone." This statement can be replace by making a list of the advantages of being alone. Some are:

1. I have time to do things I want to do.
2. I have time to think.
3. I can get to know the real me.
4. I can know what I need to work on.
5. I can figure out how I would like to go about working on this point.
6. If I am ever in a position where I have to live alone I know I am capable.

7. I will not put up with abuses from others out of my fear of being alone.
8. I become a more responsible person.

Whatever problem we are working on writing can be used as an effective means to turn irrational thoughts into more constructive thoughts. The more we write the better we will connect with our emotions using this method. I can keep these in a file, dated. From time to time I can compare notes. I can use these notes during times of setback. I can know my real self can do this. The real me need never hide out again. I can remind myself of the information written in my chapter on setbacks. I can do it. I have done it. I am not lonely. I used to be lonely. Today, I can be alone and not be lonely. I like being alone. I am growing.

I believe one of the most common of all mankind's mistakes is believing, "I can't be me without you." If we feel, "I need a man (woman) to be happy," we are in effect saying, "having a mate would solve all my problems." If having a mate would solve all problems then why are there so many unhappy married people? If we do not know ourselves we cannot communicate our true thoughts and feelings with others, decreasing our ability to have a successful relationship. we then have a nonrelationship or an entrapment. If we have not learned proper communication we could be adding to our problems by having a mate.

In this world there are people who are happy who are single and who are married. There are people who are unhappy. Be they single. Be they married. I can be as happy as I want to be. My circumstances do not determine my degree of happiness unless I let them. How I think about my circumstances determines how happy or unhappy I am and/or will be. All people have problems. Single people have problems. Married people have problems, different kinds of problems. With which set of problems do we best cope? Our thinking process makes the difference. Time and time again, lonely, dysfunctional people feel and express, "if only I had," in reference to a mate, a new car, a better job, a better figure, respect from others, whatever they feel will fill their void. As the whatever is attained they express, "if only I had...." in reference to how they went about attaining the whatever or in reference to another circumstance. The cycle of ingratitude and dysfunction continues. Loneliness, isolation from ourself, can only be filled with ourself.

Filling the hole or void with things outside ourselves will not make us complete. Filling the hole from outside of ourself being outerdirected, and dysfunctional has not brought about our completeness or whole self. Find our true self, our inner child, our true feelings, the ones which talked us through the things of which we were afraid. The one that says, "you can do it. I'm proud of of you."

Ironically, when I let go of the things the frightened part of me, who hid out because of my fears, faced the things I was frightened of, I the real me, took the risk, I found out what the real me is and isn't capable of doing. I found out I am capable of much more than I ever dreamed. There is no need to hide. I can do it. I have done it. I am doing it. I mess up sometimes. I have setbacks. All of which makes me normal, human, imperfect, average and free. What it does not make me is lonely.

When I am lonely I do not feel I have worth. I am not worthwhile because I am loved, because I care, I am not worthwhile because I achieve. I am not the sum total of my accomplishments. When all these exterior things are peeled away I have nothing left but me.

Writing this book does not make me worth more. It does, however, make me feel good. It has contributed to my healing. Who of us doesn't enjoy putting our creativity to work? King Solomon of Israel said, "take delight in the work of our hands." Instead of worrying about what I'm worth I can aim for satisfaction, learning, personal growth, and better communication. I can and have set realistic goals for myself. I am not lonely. I cannot be lonely when I feel growth inside of myself.

I always worried about my worth. Was I good enough? Finding my self respect brought me to the point where I would never doubt my worth. I feel satisfied. Communication has changed my entire life as well as the quality of my life. I am learning and growing. I feel good about myself. I never stopped to realize I had not given a thought to whether I was worth anything until I read in FEELING GOOD,

Set realistic goals for yourself and work toward them. I think you will find this so abundantly gratifying you'll forget all about worth.

How abundantly true. I agree with Dr. David Burns. When I am truly gratified I am not lonely.

WORTH

My worth depends not on acceptance,
my worth is not what I achieve,
my successes do not measure me,
that is what I believe.

I cannot do it perfect.
I'm not entitled
because I believe.

I am not omnipotent,
the world revolves not around me.

But when I am,
just what I am,
when I am free to be me,
then I have gained autonomy,
worth.

BEING AVERAGE

I never wanted to be average at anything. If I was good at whatever, I loved it. If I wasn't, I ignored it. Only do what you are good at. Now, I have found that being average is the light of my light. More than the light at the end of my tunnel. It is the tunnel itself. To my light I add more light. The pressure is off. That does not mean I can't excel at some things. I do excel at several things. it means I don't have to to feel worthwhile. Being average, I enjoy the things I do more. If I excel I have joy. If I don't excel I still have joy.

There is absolutely no way words can ever express the difference I feel. As I write this my averageness is extremely thankful for a word processor with a spell right feature. I consider my spelling on the low side of average. I have never been a very good speller. Since I have begun using this word processor my spelling has greatly improved. Something I thought would never happen. Sometimes when the speller beep beeps the word processor cannot even figure out what I am trying to spell. Back to my dictionary. If there's hope for me I know there is hope for all of us. We can improve on just about anything. We need not be the best at it. Let someone be better than me in this area. That's okay.

So, my short section on being average is just that average. And best of all I am pleased with it. Because I am pleased with myself, I am not lonely. I feel fulfilled. I have filled the void in me, with ME!

TRUE AUTONOMY

Autonomy is defined as independence. True independence is not stiff necked, inflexible or disconnected from the rest of the world. We have nothing to prove. We need not be stiff necked in order to show we can make it in the real world. Being disconnected of dysfunctional was our old way of living, with much hard work and a keen interest in self improvement we have worked, prayed, and sometimes glided along the road of recovery.

True autonomy is joy of heart, true completeness, the ability to be innerdirected, being a unique and precious self, one I was born to be. Our joy is knowing who we are, what makes us tick, how to disprove an attitude, our joy is the foundation of our autonomy. Being autonomous allows me to be and act in a legitimate, original, and unique way. I act not react to situations and other peoples actions or reactions in a way I prefer to act. Each time I am able not to react to their reaction I empower myself to be my real self, autonomous.

Our past self fulfilling prophecies were linked to our negative self image. We are putting into action the things we have learned about functionality. In this process we can establish what will be for us a positive self fulfilling prophecy. I can in order to begin my positive self fulfilling prophecy;

1. realize areas where I want personal improvement.
2. speak with functional persons.
3. Ask for positive feedback.
4. Give myself credit for the things I did right.
5. Make a list of things do right.
6. Acknowledge guilt, earned and unearned.
7. Dissipate earned guilt by making appropriate changes in our actions.
8. Let our change actions change our thinking process. Soon it feels good.
9. Dissipate unearned guilt by separating baggage appropriately.
10. Make a personal bill of rights.

Ridding ourselves of unearned guilt is accomplished by;

1. eliminating should from our vocabulary. Anytime we find ourselves saying should we need to stop and rephrase our statement in a positive way.

2. Write a declaration of self esteem. This will be our process of giving to ourselves credit for what we have done right and improvement even in areas we are still working on.

3. Read our positive affirmations out loud each day. Verbal recognition implants deeper into our subconscious new positive messages.

4. Accept compliments, simply say thank you. Let the goodness of their praise seep through your body members by taking a slow deep breath. Feel the goodness of

praise.

5. Give compliments. Return the favor. Give a compliment. We will not be mushy to say to another, "good job," or , "what a nice thought."

6. Make a do list not a do tomorrow list. My endless do tomorrow list was directly connected to , I am good enough if I can do enough. I now can set more realistic goals for myself within the course of one day. Generally I make a Do List. I do what is first priority, check it off the list, add to the list whatever new comes up and except the reality that my do list will never get done. Every once in a while I find myself getting irritable and not knowing why. I'll sit done to my desk and start to work then I realize I've been making a Do Tomorrow list for several days. Scratch that. Do what I can, settle down, take a deep cleansing breath, enjoy the work I set out to enjoy.

7. Don't be afraid to feel our guilt. Learn to say No even if we feel guilty. What have we got to lose. We do not say no, we resent, we feel guilty. We have nothing to lose by saying no and feeling guilty. We already feel guilty. Say no. Feel your guilt. Good news. This kind of guilt dissipates as we find our life getting easier.

8. Make a list of things you do right. Empower yourself. I must acknowledge

my strengths to have power to change the things about myself I do not like. When I feel good about myself I empower myself to change.

9. Use negative events for a statement of growth. We have learned to start saying, "The next time I will," instead of should thinking. The negative event that occurred can teach me only when enormous amounts of guilt do not block out the lesson I may need to learn.

10. Do not offer explanation unless you want to. My anger told me, "someone is attempting to guilt trip me in this situation." My reply was, "I will not offer an explanation if I feel guilty. If I feel it is unearned guilt. If feeling guilty do not offer an explanation. This is the time we want most to do so. Offering an explanation is our way of saying, "I am good enough," to ourselves and reaching out for their approval. Approval seeking is greatly lessened as we do not offer an explanation. Simply say, "I'm late, let's get started." Sometimes I say, "I'm sorry, I'm late can we get started." Some suggest not offering the apology. I offer the apology as my latest may have unconvinced others. It may or may not be my fault I am late. Explanations only make our appointment run longer. Let's get started.

11. Readjust unrealistic expectations, from myself and others. Becoming more functional, dancing with grace, is becoming more realistic. We more readily acknowledge our limitations. Be it how much we can achieve in one day, how important we are to this project, or our place in this universe. I am but a speck of dust in the realm of things. I am not more important than anyone else. I am not less important than anyone else.

12. Redefine emotion words- strong, tough, weakness, tears. Maybe I'm strong enough because I cry. It is found that cancer patients that are able to grieve have a higher recovery rate than those who repress their feelings. Families than grieve together heal together. Our definitions came from dysfunction. Let's redefine them in functional terms.

13. Don't fix other. When you feel like fixing hold off. When we first stop fixing we will still want to fix. This will pass as we find the joy of a life that is not burdened down with the problems of others while still caring about others. Refer back to information about three levels of detachment.

14. Don't take responsibility for their feelings. In a situation where I feel that no matter what I do someone will be hurt I tell the truth as kind as possible. Truth may cause pain but truth does no lasting harm. Lies harm, hurt, manipulate and use others.

15. Any emotion is okay to know we have it. If it is negative I can now change it. If it is positive pat myself on the back.

16. Remind myself I am not selfish. I empower myself, raise my self esteem. I now have the power to change my negative qualities. Compliment myself. I am not selfish or arrogant to think well of myself. When I think well of myself I do not think I am better than others nor do I think I am less than others. I think all persons were created equal by God.

When others disapproved we feared this would mean still others would disapprove. They disapprove = others will disapprove. NOT SO! There are ten million other people on this earth. Surly some others will approve. We empower ourselves when we refuse to give others the power to devaluate us. True Autonomy is based around our boundaries. We set and enforce boundaries as we become convinced we have the human right to boundaries. The right to think and feel differently than others. Our bill of right may include;

1. The right to be treated with respect.
2. The right to have my own feelings and opinions.
3. The right to express my feelings and opinions.
4. The right to be listened to and to be taken seriously.
5. The right to say no.

6. The right to include fun in my life.
7. The right to ask for what I need.
8. The right to ask for information I need from professionals.
9. The right to get the quality I have paid for.
10. The right to make mistakes.
11. The right to choose not to assert myself.
12. The right to have communication from those I love.
13. The right to be angry.
14. The right to be average.
15. The right to rest. The right to have imitations.

True autonomy stems from our ability to detach from dysfunctional systems and people. True autonomy acknowledges our limitations. Boundaries, detachment, and limitations are interwoven to equal US!

Establishing our right to autonomy, our level of functionality, can be aided by;

1. Making a list of each human emotion. Describe what each feeling does to you. These will be your negative aspects of that feeling. Now make a list of things this feeling does for you. This list will be positive aspects resulting from this particular feeling. Anger is almost always the first feeling others discuss. My joy is knowing almost every thing I learned in my process or recovery, each step I took toward being more functional, was in some way due to a new realization, which occurred to me because of anger on my part.

2. Recount my personal bill of rights.

3. Read Positive affirmations daily. Positive affirmations are;

I am okay.
I am adequate.

I am worthwhile.

I am special.

I am one of a kind. Oh Goodie!

I am precious.

I belong-I am a part of the universe.

I have great potential.

I am of immense value.

I enjoy being me. I truly do.

I have a zest for living.

I feel warn and happy toward myself.

I approve of myself.

I feel warm and friendly toward others. I need others in a healthy way. I am connected to others not dependent on their approval.

I can let others reject me without feeling hurt.

I look forward to new experiences. These keep me ever aware that I am growing and learning, life is exciting.

I see my mistakes as an opportunity for growing.

Each decision I make is at that moment my best decision. It is the best I could do with the information I was aware of.

I do my own thinking and learn from my own mistakes.

I am a responsible person.

I willingly accept the consequences of my own behavior.

I accept compliments without embarrassment.

I am free to express anger, joy, resentment, or love.

I accept criticism as information for my growing.

I am free. Free from the affects of dysfunction.

I am happy when others achieve. I am happy when I achieve.

I have the right to be me.

No one can be me like I can. I am the best me there is.

I am good company. I have worthwhile things to say. So do they.

I make myself happy. No one else can.

I am my own best friend.

I deserve to be trusted. I trust myself.

I deserve respect. I respect myself.

I deserve pleasure. I please myself.

I deserve love. I love myself.

I think positive thoughts. They are healthy for me.

I avoid negative thoughts. They are harmful to me.

I am filled with inner calmness and serenity.

I breather deeply and enjoy the feelings of relaxation.

I am primarily responsible for my own emotional well-being.

I share myself, my talents, my life with others.

I except miracles. Powers greater than myself perform miracles in my life each and every day.

I see the world as friendly to me.

I am a thankful person. I have always been thankful. I found reasons to be thankful among the worst of conditions.

I appreciate what others do for me without keeping track of who does more for whom.

I enjoy being alone without feeling lonely. I enjoy my thinking space. This is an important aspect of me.

I treasure the future.

I hope for the best.

4. Write a declaration of self esteem.

5. Continue to separate baggage.

6. Continue to readjust unrealistic expectations.

7. Take in as much information as possible to aid your ability to continue giving yourself credit in the areas in which you have improved.

8. Communicate your feelings in every situation possible.

9. Let important others know you expect accurate communication from them. You will probably see at least some improvement.

All of the above are steps we take to become more autonomous. We are becoming truly what we are. What we have become due to our genetics, our history, how we originally reacted to our history, and taking in new information that has allowed us to sort the things that have happened to us in this journey we call life. We are coming to a healthy state called autonomy. Autonomy means;

1. Addiction to old compulsive behaviors is no longer an issue. Very occasionally a temptation to act according to our old ways will come my way but I know how to control my impulses.

2. I understand how I benefit from long term goals. I motivate myself to work toward long term goals by setting mini goals along the way. This can be compared to a football field. We are working our way toward the goal seeing along the way the different yard lines we have passed. If we get knocked down or drug backwards we get up again, look toward our goal, and run in that direction.

3. I understand what keeps me emotionally healthy. I understand how I use recovery information and twelve step programs, reading material, feedback from others, all put together in my own unique way. A way that benefits me. This is my recovery. I have discovered through my process of recovery what works and does not work for me.

4. My recovery and autonomy are a result of honesty with others and myself. My life has become the joy of recovery not the agony of dysfunction. I need not deny to myself how I feel.

5. I feel effective in my everyday life. I have attained accurate communication skills. As I reach out to attain other goals in my life I am not nearly as afraid to learn whatever skills I need to attain those goals. Seldom do I shake and cry saying, "I can't do this." I learned through all my, "I can't do this's," that I always got up and started doing. Now when I feel nervous I know it is now an indication of whether or not I can or cannot do this. It is only an indictor of feelings that accompany something new.

6. I recognize change is exciting, fun, challenging, and inevitable. Change is nothing to fear. Change is an opportunity to grow. Disappointment can be used to earn and grow. Disappointment can lead me to releasing unrealistic expectations.

7. My problems may cause me frustration but not usually beyond solving. My solution my be step one. I am powerless over...... Seeing what I can change, what I cannot, and the insight to know the difference. I need not revert to compulsive dysfunctional behaviors to solve my problems.

8. My emotions, whatever they may be, are all normal. They are generally easy to handle. When I look back I find it almost unbelievable this was ever a problem. My feelings are indictors of my needs. Listen to them as they are my friends.

9. Self awareness: is my autonomy. I know myself well. I know what I want, why I want it. I know what I feel and why I feel it. I am my own best friend. No guilt is attacked to being my own best friend. No guilt for my feelings. I am the most important person in my life. Without me there is no my life.

All of the above are a direct result of learning the following skills;

effective communication
risk taking
problem solving

coping with my failures
facing pain
learning from my life
forgiving myself and others
independent behavior

True autonomy is not based on needing therapy on a regular bases for any length of time. Nor is it dependent on remaining part of any twelve step group for years running. Autonomy is learning the art of balance. We can go to any appropriate source for information we may need to sort through and cope with any existing problem. However, in general we feel strong enough, capable enough, we communication well the majority of the time to carry out our dealings with others and ourselves in a functional way without being dependent on a group to remind us we need to care for ourselves.

As was briefly discussed in a previous chapter we can use any therapy or twelve step group as our security or substitute family, where we receive love and emotional support, like we would hope to receive from a family but didn't. While twelve step programs are a vital support system and a necessary healing tool to truly heal we must press on beyond the group as we would have pressed on beyond the needing of approval from family if we had roots in a functional family. In the dysfunctional family we locked into needing their approval thus we stayed dysfunctional. If we lock into needing the group to function we have only replaced our original family with a group that will keep us as dysfunctional unless we learn to move beyond the needs of the group. This is about our autonomy not group autonomy.

Twelve step groups play a vital role in our healing process. It is one thing to have a therapist tell you what you think and feel are normal and another more strengthening thing to hear a room full of people express in many different ways everything you have thought and felt throughout your life. Validation to the max. As good as this is we need to continue our growth process.

The therapist I saw mentioned to me several times to be careful not to become too dependent on the group. At the time I really did not understand what he meant. I would hear people within the group talk about going to therapy seven years being in the group for ten years. I was beginning to think, I don't want to do this all my life. At that point in time I became aware that I was getting uncomfortable in the group. I did not as yet know why. What I did know was that I could not see myself going to group all my life. Soon I would become aware of what my discomfort was. I found myself angry when members of the Alanon group said things to myself and another that I knew were very dysfunctional. I addressed the fact that the problem was not alcohol the alcohol was only the symptom of the real problem; dysfunction and abuse. Members of long standing far longer than I flared with angry that I would address an issue other than alcohol. After one meeting I was told I must get rid of my anger. I did not go back. I found I was handling my life in a very functional way and I also found that I was not dependent on the group. I began to think, write, and talk about being beyond recovery. I said to my husband, "I don't think it is true that I need say I am recovering for the rest of my life. If I have an occasional slip it only puts me in the realm of normal humans everywhere. I do not need to go to a meeting to find out how to get back on track." Some time later while going through a particularly rough time I visited the Codependents Anonymous group I had attended. When I started to speak I was interrupted by an older man who said, "You did not say, 'I am a codependent, that is what this meeting is for.'" My reply, "I attended this meeting for almost two years. I came tonight as I needed feedback but instead I would like to say, I am not codependent. I have worked through my issues. Things that used to be issues no longer are. I have healthy relationships and good communication within those relationships. I need to state what I feel in the way that is comfortable to me. I am glad I came tonight because I have learned about myself. I have learned I am not codependent. I suppose I will testify to the true joy of step twelve." I then talked about a current situation in brief. Then followed with, "So, tonight I am very nervous. That is why I came, to clam down. I realize that I am nervous because I have not detached to the extent I need to for my calmness. But I handled this difficult situation totally functionally and with out guilt. I can proudly say I am no longer codependent." I was the last to speak. The group applauded. After the meeting many met me with hugs and kisses. Some old friends from the group said, "You won't be back will you?" "NO!" and most smiled, laughed, hugged, kissed and wished me well. Almost a year later I went to see my original therapist. Towards the end of the discussion he asked me if a still went to group. I said, "No, I outgrew the group. I'm beyond that." It felt good.

While twelve step groups are a soothing ointment for our wounds they are not the whole cure. They are part of our process. The major fault is that each particular group addresses their problem area. (i.e. Alcohol). But unless the issues that brought a person to use alcohol are addressed the real cause of their problems lies festering below the surface. Waiting to erupt. Which explains why AA says they are always only one drink away from slipping back into their old life style. True autonomy is accomplished by addressing the real problem that of chronic low self esteem. When we address the reasons why we have low self esteem and how we feel and felt about what happened at different times of our life we peel away layers of inconfidence, one after another till we reach our core, our true self. I believe the exact moment in time we are hit with connecting with our core and what I am is a moment in time we shall cherish all our life. This is how it worked for me. I addressed a major issue in therapy and left there on cloud nine. I would say 90% of my shame was gone that day. Soon I would begin to read. "Okay." I 'd say. Over and over as I began to see how the pieces fit. This information was chipping away at what shame was left. I began to write Profile of Abuse. And as I neared the end of John Bradshaw's Bradshaw on the Family I flew out of the chair screaming, "Harry, Harry, this is it. This is me." I did not know this was what therapy calls finding your true self. I did not know I was looking for me. But from that point on I still had a lot of work to do. Okay my shame base was gone but now it was time to learn new skills. Therapy would not be near so much about dumping my shame as it was learning that because I am angry I am not having a setback. I am only human. I will at times be angry. Therapy would be about facing how scared I was now. Although I never voiced how scared I was. My true self had never before gotten approval. I feared my marriage was headed for divorce court. Therapy would be about saying, "I think, I want, I need, I feel." Therapy would direct itself to address some marriage issues, in which my husband as well as myself would learn better communication skills. Therapy would be about learning to fight fair, learning verbal judo, and how to handle difficult people. And from time to time therapy would be a dump session for my general overall sadness when I was being to hard on myself thinking I would never get this right. Then we agreed that I should come to therapy on an as needed bases. This turned out to be a once a month thing. Recently I realized what was happening at the time was that whenever I was churning around very strong feelings I would feel I needed help. Someone help me. I felt as though I could not do this. In essence I was being too hard on myself for feelings that every person has when they feel they have been treated unfairly or when we feel betrayed or when our defenseless babies or grand babies or hurt and abused through the cruelty of a mad world. But through it all I was learning. Sometimes I thought all I did was dump. What I really did was to learn that I was figuring out the answers. I was strong enough to say, "Help me." I was strong enough to cry. I was strong enough to grieve. I was strong enough to be angry, sad, ambivalent, overwhelmed, hurt and any other human emotion I needed to feel. I was strong enough to know what I felt. Then one day as I sat at my office desk facing a tremendous new challenge of a new business feeling overwhelmed and crying, shaking and saying, "I can't do this. I can't do this. I'm just not smart enough in this area. I don't get it. I can't do this." My husband walked up put his arms around me and held me while I cried into his stomach. As I began to calm down he said, "Honey, do you know what you do?" I nodded negatively. He said, "I see you do this to yourself. Every time you hit a new stage I watch you shake and cry and say you can't do it. Then when you get done crying you get right up and do what it is you just said you can't do. You're too hard on yourself." What blessed words I heard. Just the perfect thing to say. "You are right. I do." As I recall that was my last major anxiety attack. Now when I start to feel overwhelmed I stop, take a slow breath in, let it out as slow and cleansing as I possibly can and say, "Okay Dee Frances what do you want to do first? Okay I don't get it. I can't get everything. Let's look at that again." Sometimes I must read each sentence of these new instructions over and over again working through each phrase and rewording it in my words. Okay now I get it. This helped me to learn something new about myself. When I was in high school I was in advance classes in all subjects except Math. I never felt like I belonged there. I would spend 5-6 hours a night on homework whereas other children said they spent about an hour. I would read directions over and over again breaking down each phrase until I could piece together in my mind what this meant to me. I thought they had made a big mistake putting me in these classes and I was the one to pay the price. I worked very hard for every grade I received. In reference to today I learned there are different modes of learning. Visual, audio, tactile, and imaginative in differing degrees. I am an auditory-tactile learner. An auditory learner feels they have learned a new skill when they can explain it to someone else. A tactile learner needs to feel and touch what they are walking through. For this combination what could I do better for myself than to write? To explain to other and learn what I have learned. To feel the emotions I feel as I explain it. To touch the keys of my computer as I explain what I have learned to another. So welcome to the world Dee Frances who feels great joy with my new explanation. What does this have to do with, Can I have this dance? Everything. It changed my view of myself. I am not dense because I have a hard time with written directions involving learning a new skill. I can recognize my learning modes. I can word things so that I understand that I understand. I can work my way through new dance steps, a new computer skills, a new book distributor. I can reword it back to myself and know, "I got it." I can touch it and taste. I can dance. I can sing. I can do most anything. I can write a book and share my thoughts with you. Thoughts that have helped me to continue to grow more functional and more confident ever knowing that I will have times of doubt, times when I feel overwhelmed, times when I want someone to carry my load or at least help me up while I carry my load. I can do all these things and dance my dance. Walk my way through the steps. Learn my dance until I am satisfied with my skill, grace, and pace.

In closing I would like to repeat the statement in this book that I believe to be the synopsis of breaking the cycle of dysfunction. It is:

We are starting to understand ourselves, other people and the world of communication. Communication is the link between our true self and the rest of the world. When we have accurate communication and know how to use it in everyday situations we are becoming functional. Recently I read that it is better to seek to understand rather that to be understood. This I feel is accurate. This is not the dysfunction of caring more about others than myself but the function of connecting with the rest of the universe. here again is a paradox of recovery. When I seek to be understood chances are-I don't receive it. When I seek to understand others chances are-I receive understanding. When I understand others I will be understood to a greater degree. What will be understood about myself is whatever is my degree of empathy, love, and genuine caring. What will be understood about myself is my level of love for my God and my fellow man.

Add onto the above rhetorical our being part of our core, our natural self. I must conclude with we have broken the cycle of dysfunction. We are dancing to the music of our core, our real self. We have learned the art of leading, the art of following, the value of timing. We have learned grace and pose, dignity instead of family shame. We can dance our heart out. Be it a waltz, a two step, or the jitter bug, or any combination of the above. None of us are all one but perhaps we are all all of the above. We are being what we truly are. We have given up fear of what others think. We have learned that repressing our feelings is a way of feeling we can control what others think of us. We have learned the true art of being functional is: I can take care of me without hurting you. And with that in mind we can ask or answer the following questions. Can I have this dance? Can we dance for the rest of our lives?

REVIEW

SECTION

BIBLIOGRAPHYOPHY

52 Ways To Reduce Stress In Your Life by Connie Neal c 1993 published by Nelson Publishers of Nashville

52 Simple Ways To Tell Your Child "I Love You" by Jan Dargatz c1991 published by Nelson Publishers of Nashville

An Adult Child's Guide To What's "Normal" by John Friel, PhD. & Linda Friel, M.A. c 1990 Published by Health Communications of Florida

Don't Talk, Don't Trust, Don't Feel by Robert A. Becker PhD c 1991 Published by Health Communications of Florida

Transforming The Codependent Woman by Sandy Bierig c 1991 Published by Health Communications

Bradshaw On: The Family by John Bradshaw c 1988 Published by Health Communications

Light His Fire by Ellen Kreidman c 1991 Published by Dell Publishing of New York

Light Her Fire by Ellen Kreidman c 1989 Published by Dell Publishing of New York

Listen Up: Hear What's Really Being Said by Jim Dugger c 1991 Published by National Press Publications

Parenting: Ward And June Don't Live Here Anymore by Jim Dugger c 1991 published by National Press Publications

Real Men Don't Vacuum by S.J.. GELB Ph.D. c 1991 Published by National Press Publications

Assertiveness: Get What You Want Without Being Pushy by Cal LeMon c1990 Published by National Press Publications

Little Miss Perfect by Megan LeBoutillier c 1987 Published by Ballantine Books of New York

You Just Don't Understand, Women And Men In Conversation by Deborah Tannen, PhD. c 1990 Published by Ballantine Books of New York

I'm Ok- You're Ok by Thomas A. Harris M.D. c 1963 Published by Harper and Row of New York

Men Are From Mars, Women Are From Venus by John Gray, PhD. c 1992 Published by Harper Collins

Beginning to Heal by Ellen Bass and Laura Davis c 1993 Published by Harper Perennial

Codependent No More by Melody Beattie c 1987 Published by Harper/HAZELDEN of San Francisco

Beyond Codependency by Melody Beattie c1989 Published by Harper/HAZELDEN of San Francisco

The Courage to Heal by Ellen Bass and Laura Davis c 1988 Published by Harper Perennial

For Your Own Good by Alice Miller c 1990 Published by The Noonday Press of New York

Adult Children of Abusive Parents by Steven Farmer c 1989 Published by Comtemporary Books of Chicago

Codependent' Guide to the Twelve Steps by Melody Beattie c 1990 Published by Prentice Hall Press of New York

How To Forgive When You Don't Know How by Jacqui Bishop, M.S. & Mary Grunte, R.N. c 1993 Published by Station Hill Press

God's Psychiatry by Charles L. Allen c 1953 Published by Power Books of Tarrytown, New York

The 12 Steps For Adult Children c 1987 written and published by the staff of Recovery Publications

A Time To Heal by Timmen L. Cermak, M.D. c 1989 Published by Avon Books

Homecoming by John Bradshaw c 1990 Published by Bantam Books

A Reason to Live Edited by Melody Beattie c 1989 Published by Tyndale House Publishers, Inc. of Wheaton Ill

Mind and Mood by Dr. Robert Curtis c 1986 Published by Charles Scribner's Sons of New York

The Real Thirteenth Step by Tina Tessina, PhD. c 1991 by Jeremy P. Tarcher/ Perigee Books of New York

All I Really Need To Know I Learned In Kindergarten by Robert Fulghum c 1988 Published by Ivy Books of New York

Feeling Good by David D. Burns, M.D. c 1980 Published by New American Library of New York

The Complete Guide to Your Emotions and Your Health by Emrika and the editors of Prevention Magazine c 1986

Roget's International Thesaurus Fourth Edition by Harper & Row c 1997

Student Handbook including Webster's New World Dictionary Volume Two c 1982 by Simon & Schuester

The Layman's Parallel Bible by Zondervanb Bible Publishers of Grand Rapids, Michigan c 1973

ANGER - IN REVIEW

1. What is the meaning of outerdirected?
2. How do we find out how to use our anger to grow?
3. What common factors are there between this situation and situations of our past?
4. What do we feel immediately before we are aware of our anger?
5. What are we afraid of?
6. Is conflict always negative?
7. Name two basic styles of conflict.
8. How can we tell the difference in types of conflict?
9. How can I use conflict to grow?

REVIEW

1. What are three different ways to handle anger?
2. What does each method do to you and for you?
3. Which do you feel is most appropriate?
4. What is the difference between talking yourself out of anger and talking your way through your anger?
5. In the process of working through anger, what are some things each of us can do to come to understand the bottom line premise of why we are angry?
6. What are some benefits of processing our anger?
7. What is the difference between assertive and aggressive?
8. When there is a need to confront the person I am upset with what is meant by fighting with dignity?
9. What is conflict?
10. List three factors that cause conflict.
11. List five stages of conflict resolution.
12. What is negotiation?
13. When both sides give in a little to reach a solution, what are they doing?

REVIEW TO LISTENING EFFECTIVELY SKILLS

Listen with empathy.

Listen nonjudgmentally.

Speak in I messages showing you understand.

Express feeling messages to help the other to be able to say what they need to say.

Use active I messages.

Ask open ended questions.

Respond to the behavior or idea not the person.

Respond in the present tense.

Respond by describing, not evaluating.

Respond nonjudgmentally.

Don't force someone to share their feelings.

Use reflective listening to highlight important issues.

Respond as accurately as you can.

Respond as honestly as you can.

Reflect back positive and pleasant feelings.

Don't expect to get active listening perfect.

If the problem is to big for both of you seek expert advice.

REVIEW TO LESSENING STRESSFUL SITUATIONS

1. Not letting others irritate you. Sometime they are deliberately trying to provoke you. You can take your sail out of their wind.

2. Focus on the positive. This may truly not bother you when you look for the positive.

3. Change the subject to something constructive. Lighten up the situation.

4. Take a personal stand against serious conflict, especially physical. Realize this harms people. Work for nonviolent resolutions.

5. Don't let people intimidate you or bully you into fighting. You can show your strength by doing what you want to do, not what others want or try to control you into doing.

6. Simply walk away. We can say, "Let's talk later when we are calm."

REVIEW

1. How can learning to handle disagreements strengthen relationships?
2. What types of factors cause conflict?
3. What are the stages of conflict?
4. What skills can you use to resolve conflict?
5. How many issues should be addressed at one time?
6. What is respect?
7. Can conflict be prevented?
8. How can we reduce conflict?
9. What is compromise?
10. Why is listening so important to conflict resolution?

11. What is more important a person's words or his body language?
12. What types of things cause barriers to conflict resolution?
13. What might happen if a person represses his anger for too long a period of time?
14. Why must some people win the argument?

BOOKS BY DEE FRANCES

Let's Communicate, Breaking the Cycle of Non- Communication is rich with information and easy-to-understand examples for healthy living. the reader can identify with an author who has 'been there.' $24.95

Profile of Abuse - The theme of which is; I can take care of me without hurting you. Assertive not aggressive without a problem. $12 OR PROOFING COPY $6.

Positive Thinking Easier Than You Think- 261 affirmations to lift us up and out of the negativities. A positive mental handle to grab on to. $9.95

Inspirational Verses - Journal - Each page is topped with an upbuilding verse with room for the reader to respond, pro or con. $10.

Reflections of a Time- poetry about life and the beauty that encompasses us by our surrounding universe. $8.95

A Tribute to a Grandmother poetry $7 Edited by Dee Frances the published works of Dee's grandmothers Eunice Boyd Hackward.

How to Poetry! A Workbook A fun activity book to improve verse writting. Great for all newcomers to poetry, those with writers block, and children learning about poetry. $8

Poems and Growth, from me to me. Personal growth and recovery expressed in poem. Poems about the agony of codependency and the joy of recovery. $ 8.95

Flying High Through Poetry - The Music of Life an DDDD Publications 1997 anthology.

What is Poetry? Columns from A Poemazine's first year. $5

A Journal of Growth, A Workbook - Live in the Now. Learn how to handle this problem today, not the 182 problems that this reminds us of. Decide for yourself which is easier, which is best for you. $12.95

How To Stay In Love - probably one of the most asked questions ever. We need not climb the highest mountain, or swim the deepest sea for me to stay in love with you and you to stay in love with me. An antidote to 101 ways to screw up your relationship. $5.95

Relationship Compatibility - Discover and remedy weak relationship areas by Dee Frances. Invaluable to those approaching the subject of marriage. But don't forget no matter the length of the marriage we all have shortcomings therefore our relationships do too. $8

Personal Growth in a Nutshell- Quick & Easy $10 You'll laugh and cry at this wonderful book, quick to read, easy to apply.

Thirteen Blessings of the Twelve Steps - count the blessings we receive as we work our way through the twelve steps. There were at least thirteen sets of blessings that came my way. Bringing me to the grand conclusion of....... $12.95

In the Mid of Night - poetry. Dee's poetry which allowed her to work through feelings that grew from a dysfunctional family background. Other poetry is for the pure enjoyment of being alive and living our lives to know we make a difference in this universe. $12.95

POET IN MOTION - released August 96. Poetry for fun, poetry for personal growth, poetry from the brush of Dee Frances. "My artist brush with hairs of words is strung," is one of Dee's favorite expressions. You too will delight in her words. Laugh your way through the pocm E - MAIL IT TO ME. $8.95

1475 Conclusions of a Healing Codependent - Each new conclusion we draw changes the person we are at least to some degree. Perhaps changes that will bring a more postive, happier self. $9.95

KIDS BOOKS

Pink Milk Sea: My First Self Esteem Reader $5

I Live with My Grandma children today live in a different world than 20 years ago. More and more chidlren are being raised by grandparents. Additonally many mothers work from home. This great book explains today's world to the delight of any child. $10

SHORT STORIES, PUZZLES & MORE - COMPILATION OF AUTHORS - $10

MORE FOR KIDS

STORYZINE - a monthly newsletter - short stories, puzzles, neat facts, animal facts, games, and jokes. A one year subscription is $25. Subscribe with a friend and each saves $5.

ORDER ANY OF THESE BOOKS FOR YOURSELF, YOUR FAMILY, AND YOUR FRIENDS Send check or money order to: DDDD Publications PO Box 140081 St Louis Mo 63114

Include cost of book and/or books and $4.00 S & H

TRIFOLD &/OR REPORTS BY DEE FRANCES
COST $3 EACH OR 4 FOR $10

ESTABLISHING A GRATITUDE CYCLE
LOVE IS . . .
IT'S CONTROL WHEN. . ..
FRIENDS - WHAT MEN CAN TEACH WOMEN
AFTER RAPE - WHAT TO DO
AFTER THE LOSS OF A CHILD
EVERYTHING I NEEDED TO KNOW - I HAD TO FIGURE OUT
MY SELF ESTEEM VERSES MY WEIGHT
FOUR STAGES OF ANY RELATIONSHIP
TEARS - BENEFICIAL TO ALL
I'M NOT PERFECT - A GUIDE FOR PARENTS
I'M NOT PERFECT - A GUIDE FOR RELATIONSHIPS
BECOMING SOLUTION ORIENTED - A POSITIVE CYCLE
5 WAYS TO IMPROVE CONFIDENCE
VICTIM TO VICTOR
PINPOINTING DEPRESSION
WHEN I'M FUNTIONAL
A SALUTE TO THE ACCOMPLISHEMENTS OF WOMEN
FEMALE TREATMENT VERSES MALE MUST BE DIFFERERENT FOR MOST
EFFECTIVE CARE - chemical addiction
12 WAYS TO PREVENT BURNOUT
SOMETHING GREW- THE TRUE ME
TIPS FOR THE BACK TO SCHOOL WOMAN
A WOMAN'S ROLE?
CONFUSED - ANGRY- FRUSTRATED AND FUNCTIONAL
A LESSON FOR MOM
FUNCTIONAL VERSES DYSFUNCTIONAL
LOVING HELP OR CONTROL WHICH
KIDS CHORES- WHAT CHORES? - WHAT AGE?
ALCOHOL - SIGNS OF A PROBLEM
SEXUAL HARASSMENT - WHAT IS IT?
WHAT IS HUMAN IMPERFECTION?- WHAT IS ABUSE?
SECRETS TO A GOOD NIGHT'S SLEEP
KID'S PRIVACY?
THE X THAT MAKES THE DIFFERNCE
CHRISTIAN DYSFUNCTION DIFFERS FROM IMMORALITY
THE ABC'S OF CHILD REARING
THE IMPORTANCE OF GRANDPARENTS
PICKING A QUALITY DAY CARE
UNDERSTANDING PRESCHOOL THINKING
YOUR CHILD AND KINDERGARTEN
HELPING KIDS OVERCOME THEIR FEARS
LOVE THEN - DON'T SPOIL THELM
4 STEPS TO TEACHING PATIENCE
RAISING KIDS THAT CARE - IN VIOLENT TIMES
DESTRESSING YOUR MARRIAGE
PICKING A LOYAL CONFIDANT
5 STEPS TO LESSENING STRESS
MASTERING YOUR NERVES

NOTICING AND HELPING A CHILD WITH DEPRESSION
RECOGNIZING A.D.D.
10 DISCIPLINE MISTAKES
DAD IS IMPORTANT WITH YOUR CHILD
EFFECTS OF TEENAGE SEX
FOR THE FAMILY WHO DIDN'T ABUSE
7 PUBLIC SPEAKING MISTAKES
DE-BRATING YOUR CHILD

UPCOMING BOOKS BY DDDD PUBLICATIONS

CRAFTING POETRY, The How To's....... by Dee Frances The easiest explaination of the complicated craft of poetry in print. $15 ISBN 1-885519-18-4

PUT A SMILE ON YOUR FACE, It's Time to Get Happy by Dee Frances Be the best that you can be. Instant easy ways to improve your attitude. Learn more effective ways to handle negaholics, stressful times, anxiety attacks, chronic pain, and chronic illness. $24.95

SMALL CHANGE by Floriana Hall One woman's person account of growing up in the depression. Flo's account is written for the grade school level in order to children to connect with older person with greater levels of understanding. ISBN 1-885519-04-4 $12

SANDS OF RYHME by Floriana Hall Poetry 1-885519-07-9

OH, COULDN'T IT, A Novella and Other Writings by F.S. Eagle. Mr. Eagle's account of life of campus during unsettlings times. ISBN 1-885519-15-X $12

BLACK IS NOT A COLOR by Mary Douglas Poetry. 1-885519-16-8 $10

ONE ROSE by Mary Douglas Poetry 1-885519-17-6

GLIMPES OF GOLDEN MOUNTAIN by Mike Nolan. Poetry. ISBN $10